effective learning & teaching in MEDICAL, DENTAL & VETERINARY EDUCATION

Edited by john sweet, sharon huttly & ian taylor

ilt
the institute for learning and teaching in higher education

THE TIMES HIGHER EDUCATION SUPPLEMENT

Routledge
Taylor & Francis Group
LONDON AND NEW YORK

First published in 2003 by Kogan Page Limited

Published 2016 by Routledge
2 Park Square, Milton Park, Abingdon, Oxfordshire OX14 4RN
711 Third Avenue, New York, NY 10017

First issued in hardback 2016

Routledge is an imprint of the Taylor and Francis Group, an informa business

ISBN 13: 978-1-138-15134-5 (hbk)
ISBN 13: 978-0-7494-3562-2 (pbk)

British Library Cataloguing-in-Publication Data

A CIP record for this book is available from the British Library.

Contents

About the editors and specialist contributors

Editors

John Sweet is a specialist in Periodontics and Lecturer at University of Wales Dental School in Cardiff. He has contributed to a range of changes in the dental curriculum at Cardiff and various interprofessional initiatives in the other schools of the University of Wales College of Medicine and is particularly interested in staff and educational developmental issues. He spent five years lecturing in the Medical Faculty of the University of the West Indies. An advocate for the ILT from its inception, he is currently Secretary for ILT Wales.

Sharon Huttly is Reader in International Child Health and Development at the London School of Hygiene and Tropical Medicine. She is also the School's Teaching Programme Director with responsibility for overseeing the delivery and strategic development of the postgraduate taught courses. She has 18 years' experience in higher education and is interested in a range of learning and teaching issues, especially those concerning international postgraduate students. She spent three months' study leave at the Institute for Learning and Teaching in Higher Education (ILT) in 2000.

Ian Taylor is Director of the Liverpool Evaluation and Assessment Unit at the University of Liverpool. He has an especial interest in work-based learning, and has worked on a range of national and regional projects, focussing on undergraduate and professional development. Current commitments include a programme, supported by the British Council, to promote off-campus learning for veterinary undergraduates in Bangladesh, and a project funded by the Learning Skills Council to promote professional development in teachers.

Specialist contributors

Stephen Brigley is Senior Lecturer in Medical Education at the University of Wales College of Medicine and has wide experience in post-compulsory education. He has published on educational issues including management ethics and learning and teaching in medicine. He directs a postgraduate certificate in medical education and has research interests in portfolio learning and cultures of learning and teaching. **George Brown** is Special Professor of Education at the University of Nottingham and Senior Tutor for the MMedSci programme in Clinical Education. He has long experience of working in dental, medical and nurse education and in academic staff development. He has conducted research and written extensively on many issues of teaching, learning and assessment.

Ronald Brown is Lecturer in Dental Technology at the Dental School of the University of the West Indies, Trinidad, and specializes in teaching the technical aspects of crown and bridge and prosthetic work to undergraduates. He started his career in the Conservation Department at Edinburgh Dental School, soon became interested in teaching and has wide-ranging experience working at Dental Schools in England, Ireland, Saudi Arabia and Papua New Guinea.

Joy Crosby is a Lecturer in Medical Education and the Curriculum Facilitator at Dundee Medical School. The undergraduate course at Dundee is renowned for its progressive approach to assessment building upon such innovations as the OSCE. Joy also has a particular interest in learner-centred modes of learning, particularly small group learning and has published guides and chapters on this topic.

John Eyers is Deputy Librarian at the London School of Hygiene & Tropical Medicine. For over 20 years he has taught information retrieval techniques to postgraduate students and, recently, at St John's Medical College, Bangalore. His particular interest lies in teaching effective database and Internet searching and critical appraisal of sources of information.

Heather Fry is Head of the Imperial College Centre for Educational Development, London. She teaches, publishes, and researches across a range of areas, including teaching, learning and assessment, especially in medical and dental education, curriculum change and course design, and policy in higher and professional education.

Michael Manogue is the Dean for Learning and Teaching in the Faculty of Medicine, Dentistry, Psychology and Health of the University of Leeds and Senior Lecturer in Restorative Dentistry in the Leeds Dental Institute. Recent research publications include empirical studies of OSCEs in Dentistry and a national survey of methods of assessment used in restorative dentistry.

Gerry Mullins is Senior Lecturer in the Adelaide Graduate Centre at the University of Adelaide. Apart from his work on postgraduate education, he has been involved in the implementation of the new Adelaide dental curriculum from the initial stages, and continues to contribute to collaborative research on the outcomes of the Adelaide dental curriculum.

Iain Robbé is Senior Lecturer in public health medicine at the University of Wales College of Medicine and Honorary Consultant to Bro Taf Health Authority. He specializes in medical and other healthcare education for both undergraduates and postgraduates. His current research interests include teaching governance and investigating how adult learners learn with their peers and facilitators in the curriculum.

Madeleine Rohlin is Professor of Oral Radiology at the Faculty of Odontology, Malmö University, Sweden. She led the team that developed the fully integrated PBL curriculum in dental education at Malmö, which started in 1990. Her main research interests are diagnostic efficacy, clinical decision-making, and collaborative learning in dentistry.

Andrew Sackville is Head of Teaching and Learning Development at Edge Hill College of Higher Education. He is programme leader for a successful multidisciplinary Postgraduate Certificate in Teaching and Learning in Clinical Practice delivered by supported online learning. His current research interests focus on the design of opportunities for interaction in online and e-learning programmes.

John Wetherell is a part-time Senior Lecturer in the Dental School and runs a busy private practice in the suburbs of Adelaide. He is particularly interested in developing the reflective aspects of student learning through student self-assessment and the use of journals of reflection.

Jeff Wilson is Senior Lecturer at the University of Wales College of Medicine and specializes in teaching Restorative and Prosthetic Dentistry in which he has 20 years' experience. He also teaches communication skills to medical undergraduates. His research interests include undergraduate education and support as well as clinical prosthetics.

Acknowedgements

We would like to thank Sally Brown, Series Editor of this series of *Effective Learning and Teaching* books and Jonathan Simpson from Kogan Page for commissioning us to edit this book, and the support given to us throughout its production. We developed the book outline and have been delighted with the enthusiasm with which the contributers have tackled their remit and augmented the original concepts. We are particularly pleased to have contributions from Scandinavia, the Caribbean and Australia in addition to those from the United Kingdom, including England, Scotland and Wales and thank them all for their efforts. We would also like to thank both students and colleagues who have provided us with food for thought and encouragement: in particular John Ackers, Jeff Wilson and Ronald Brown and John Wetherell. Finally we are indebted to Sir Kenneth Calman, President of the ILT for writing a preface.

Foreword

I am delighted to see in print this fourth volume in the *Effective Learning and Teaching* series. The editors are to be congratulated on the immense amount of hard work they have invested in putting together this important contribution to the literature on learning and teaching in medicine, dentistry and veterinary science. Teaching medicine, dentistry and veterinary science is a complex and demanding task, undertaken alongside other demanding duties and I am sure that readers will find much useful information and advice in this book as well as useful contact information and references to further reading.

The ILT is now at an important stage in its development with almost 17,000 who have applied to join the organization as we go to press, and with 125 programmes in higher education teaching and learning accredited by the ILT and a full programme of publications, activities and events on offer. Now with members in the majority on our governing council, active on all our committees and working parties and getting involved in the running of our members' forums and other events, members are increasingly taking charge of shaping and directing the policy and direction of the organization.

This book has a part to play in the ILT's mission to enhance the status of teaching, improve the experience of learning and supporting innovation in higher education. I commend it to you, whether you are an ILT member or not and welcome the contribution it makes to the higher education context.

Sally Brown
Director of Membership Services
Institute for Learning and Teaching

Preface

What is so special about teaching and learning in medicine, dentistry and veterinary medicine? What makes it different? Perhaps it is because, in common with all professional groups, the learning process occurs within the context of people, patients, clients, animal owners, who have their own values and feelings to be taken into account. It is thus impossible to consider teaching and learning in these three subjects without attention being given to this dimension.

Thus, in addition to learning the factual knowledge and skills required to master the basics of the subject and deliver care, there are also the emotional knowledge base and attitudes to consider. How do people feel about their health or their illness? How will they respond to learning the diagnosis and possible treatment? What are the issues of an ethical nature that need to be considered? Thus, the learning and the teaching must not only be student-centred, but patient-centred.

A key factor is the rapidly changing knowledge base and the need for students and practitioners to be able to deal with new problems and new solutions. The continuing and lifelong nature of the learning process is clear. The relationship with the patients is also changing as they, and the public, become more knowledgeable and aware of the implications of their health and the ways in which it might be maintained. This is a very positive aspect of the changed relationship and may become the most powerful force for changing professional practice.

The learning and teaching depend also on the selection of the students and their expectations of the course. Thus students who are problem-solvers, critical thinkers, team workers and communicators will require, and demand, a different type of curriculum, teaching methods, and assessment process.

For clinical students there is also the need to support them during the course and ensure that they have time to reflect on what they have learnt and seen. They need an opportunity to discuss their own problems with someone who can take them through what might be difficult personal issues.

For the teacher, the privilege of facilitating the learning of such a special group of students is a reward in itself. The knowledge that a graduate will be able to care for, in a professionally competent way, those who are ill and to be able to apply their factual and emotional knowledge so that patients and their families will benefit, is a proper aim to reach for.

I welcome this book as a useful contribution to our understanding of learning, teaching and assessment issues associated with these subject areas. As Chair of the rapidly growing Institute for Learning and Teaching, which is commissioning the books, I welcome the series as a means of promoting effective learning and teaching, not just among our members, but also in the wider community of learning in the UK and beyond.

Sir Kenneth C Calman
Chair of the Institute for Learning and Teaching in Higher Education

Introduction

Sharon Huttly and John Sweet

Medicine, dentistry and veterinary science are three traditional but rapidly changing professions. Like other professions they are experiencing an ever-increasing expansion in their knowledge base and their training is situated within a higher education sector that has undergone radical changes in recent decades. Although medical, dental and veterinary (MDV) education spans a significant breadth, as suggested by the formation in 1999 of the Learning and Teaching Subject Network, which placed these three areas in a single Subject Centre, there is considerable overlap in the particular features of these fields. For example, the shift from teacher-centred to learner-centred approaches in higher education has additionally had to accommodate another dimension in MDV education, namely patient-centred approaches. The change in public trust of the sciences and the professions in general is perhaps particularly manifest in these areas and today's MDV students can no longer expect the 'trust me I'm a doctor' approach to patient care to be sufficient or acceptable. Today's patients have more information available to them, are more aware of their rights and are more prepared to challenge those in whose care they might be.

MDV education has had to face these changes and modify itself accordingly. Undoubtedly more changes are ahead. Thus this book will place emphasis on what is special about student learning in medicine, dentistry and veterinary medicine and the teaching opportunities in these fields. Emphasis will also be placed on issues that are changing, so that learners and teachers can work positively with change and indeed become agents for change themselves and contribute to improvements within their own institutions. The book addresses some generic issues in higher education but looked at from an MDV perspective, each chapter gives references for general as well as specific reading on that topic.

The audience

This book is intended for both new and experienced teaching staff in MDV education. For new teachers, this book will give leads and links to new sources of outside help on the one hand, and also guidance on ways to develop and assess student learning and their own teaching on the other. Some chapters will challenge the new lecturer to start a process of self-assessment that can nurture a personal philosophy and style of teaching. Those requiring a general handbook for teaching can refer to the texts listed at the end of this chapter.

In addition, this book is designed to help established teachers who wish to develop their practice. Those who are currently using patient- and student-centred approaches in their particular field will be able to gain perspective, encouragement and stimulation from the various chapters that advocate that practice. Those who currently use more traditional teaching methods will find a range of ideas to expand their repertoire; Chapter 6 on interactive lecturing is a good place to start.

Learning from others

While medical, dental and veterinary education have many overlapping features, they have also developed in different ways and have their own distinctive features. The editors and chapter authors of this book are drawn from these three interrelated subject areas and it is hoped that their writings and experiences will offer the reader from one area new ideas for application from another. A number of authors are from outside the United Kingdom so that although the emphasis is on UK-based MDV education, and reference is made to particular UK bodies such as the General Medical Council, an international perspective is also present.

The structure

This book can be used as a dip-into handbook, as each chapter is written as a discrete entity. However, the book tells a story that can be read *in toto* or in parts. The chapters were commissioned to allow each author to expand a theme in MDV education. The underlying pragmatic philosophy of the book is that of grasping every opportunity to develop MDV education, and that whilst this involves individual teachers and students, it is best conducted collaboratively in an institution that is willing to support educational development. A hypothetical MDV educational centre is outlined in Chapter 1, based on forward-looking initiatives occurring in MDV Schools and HE generally. A more theoretical underpinning of the case for collegiality and collaborative learning within the MDV culture is outlined in Chapter 2. Despite considerable curricular changes, especially in medical education, the authors argue that MDV education cultures are not keeping pace with cultural change in society. MDV education is more a process of adapting to a new professional culture, than the imbibing of knowledge. The authors make a range of suggestions to further cultural change within MDV education. One key component is development of communication skills, for without this the link to the patient is broken (Chapter 3).

Central to the enhancement of MDV educational programmes is the concept of curriculum. This is reviewed in Chapter 4 where the author has made the case for MDV curricula that, whilst focussing on the student experience, are broadly conceived to support a patient (possibly pet owner in the case of an animal), community and other professional health care workers. Extreme curricula, where staff are over-preoccupied with the didactic delivery of knowledge, problems, breakdown of specific competence or computer use, are rejected in favour of an all-stakeholder approach. Chapter 5 details the variety and importance of aligning appropriate assessment procedures to the devised curriculum. Methods that teachers can use to facilitate learning are discussed in the three chapters, 6, 7 and 8 that follow on teaching in small and large groups and the use of information technology and online learning.

There follow three more chapters on different issues that affect student learning directly. Chapter 9 is concerned with student support; the kind of nurturing beyond narrow academic needs. Using a dental technology as an example, Chapter 10 outlines how educational theory can be applied to concepts and in educational practice in an attempt to improve the learning experience for students. Chapter 11 focusses specifically on the clinical environment and the challenges and opportunities this presents to innovative teachers. Learning from experience has a vital role to play in clinical education and is mentioned in many of the chapters. The process of developing reflective clinical practice is more formally considered in Chapter 12 with an emphasis on the use of portfolios.

Chapter 13 explores concepts of quality of clinical teaching, challenges leaders to reflect on their own teaching and looks at how this is framed by issues such as infrastructure and departmental working practices. Chapter 14 draws the book to a close by considering the latest developments in the professions and attempts to predict future trends in clinical education.

The structure of this book can also be described along the lines used as the basis for membership of the Institute for Learning and Teaching in Higher Education (the ILT), which considers professional activity in five broad areas:

- teaching and the support of learning;
- contribution to the design and planning of learning activities and/or programmes of study;
- assessment and giving feedback to learners;
- developing effective learning environments and learner support systems;
- reflective practice and personal development.

Chapters 1 to 8 address the first two of these areas. Chapter 5 takes a comprehensive look at clinical assessment and feedback to learners and these important issues are also brought to light in Chapter 10. Chapters 9 to 11 consider the fourth area of effective learning environments and learner support systems. Chapters 12 and 13 lead to the concept of reflective practice and both the development of the teacher at an individual level and the issues of concern at institutional level such as benchmarking and quality.

The final chapter, 14, attempts to build on the current changes in MDV education and to look ahead to the challenges that must be faced in the future. We see the issues contained in these chapters as addressing two of the ILT's principal aims – improving the experience of learning, and supporting innovation in higher education.

References

General texts on teaching in higher education:

Biggs, J (1999) *Teaching for quality learning at university: What the student does*, SRHE and OUP, Buckingham

Curzon, B L (2000) *Teaching in Further Education*, 5th edn, Pippin Publishing Corporation, London

Fry, H, Ketteridge, S and Marshall, S (1999) *A Handbook for Teaching and Learning in Higher Education: Enhancing Academic Practice*, Kogan Page, London

Race, P (1999) *2000 Tips for Lecturers*, Kogan Page, London

Race, P (2001) *The Lecturer's Toolkit*, 2nd edn, Kogan Page, London

1

Opportunities in medical, dental and veterinary (MDV) educational development

John Sweet

Introduction

The opportunities for learning and teaching in MDV education are immense. For a start, it is not enough for strategies to be just student-centred; they must be patient-centred as well. They must also be robust enough to enable teachers and learners to handle the various third party, individual and corporate forces that can either enhance or impinge upon the care of patients. Effective strategies often entail situated learning, which ranges from tertiary level to working within the community. The long length of the course and potentially invasive nature of treatment often dictate a favourable ratio of staff to students, which can be exploited. However, some foci in MDV education are very short of staff. The team healthcare approach at work can also be simulated in MDV education through interprofessional education and vertical integration of student years and extended into concepts of lifelong learning in postgraduate courses. Effective communication is an essential skill in MDV practice that can be taught and assessed. The practitioner needs to master a range of information technology (IT) skills and writing genres, within a multidisciplinary environment. Few fields outside the MDV world offer the possibilities of depth and range of activity, which teachers can use to nurture new reflective practitioners who, using best evidence, can attempt to treat patients optimally.

The approach in this chapter is to concentrate on how an MDV School within the university setting could utilize a centre for educational development. This complements Chapter 10, which concentrates on a lecturer's personal teaching strategy. I set out a personal view, which, firstly, tries to articulate a range of activities a centre should take in its main function as a community of staff and students. Secondly, the reader is prompted to think about their own organization, identify how learning and teaching is currently supported and to envisage what further developments might be appropriate. Fortunately, forward-thinking vice-chancellors are putting forward their own vision for the future of their universities but are also offering to be receptive to ideas especially if they provide solutions. This chapter is therefore designed to stimulate management either directly or indirectly to fund and organize educational development appropriately within their institutions. Another aim is to encourage lecturers to envisage the contribution they might make towards the organization's success. A similar but wider ranging Centre for Higher Education Development for a predominantly non-healthcare university is well documented on the World Wide Web (Coventry University, 2002).

My concept of educational development for a hypothetical MDV university includes a learning and teaching centre that can lead and nurture teaching but primarily provides a home base for a community of educators. This is a creative unit that allows the lecturer to work with the centre and so achieve more than they would working alone. This, in essence, is what teaching enhancement and educational development is about – evolving participatory collaboration, critically testing learning activities and creating credible evidence of their impact.

Functions of the centre

Communication

One of the major functions of the centre must be to improve communication and the impact of educational developments on improving the learning of students.

In an inspiring chapter, Boyer (1989) states that 'In the end, the quality of a College can be measured by the quality of communication on the campus'. This includes the relationship between MDV professional and patient (outlined in Chapter 3 in this book). As Boyer says 'the doctor who knows only disease is at a disadvantage alongside the doctor who knows as much about people as he or she does about pathological organisms'. But communication must also provide a healthy link between teachers and between teachers and students. Within the process of lifelong learning the teachers become lifelong students. Boyer would also reciprocate and say that 'we need to create a climate... in which students are teachers, too'.

Teacher development

A major thrust of the centre is to encourage educational self-development. It is clear that there cannot be curricular development without staff development, for it is the staff interactions with students, the materials they prepare and systems they put in place that deliver an environment that the students will apprehend as the educational climate (Genn, 2001).

Practical tips and useful literature

Many who teach in MDV are busy doing something else; either research or a practical clinical service commitment to patients. This can be most helpful in the teaching programme because the teacher is in a position to converse about the topic content or patient management with authority. When it comes to enhancing the learning experience of students, the busy teachers will be looking for useful teaching tips. The centre should encourage these lecturers to attend forums, to share good practice and attend both presentations and workshops geared to enhance teaching skills. The centre should also direct these lecturers to some of the very good generic books on this topic such as Fry, Ketteridge and Marshall (1999); Gibbs, Habeshaw and Habeshaw (1988) and Race (1999). Specific tips for MDV education on how to enhance lectures, small group teaching and assessment are contained in Chapters 5, 6 and 7 of this book, but throughout there is equal emphasis on educational theory, as this can inform and help deliver appropriate teaching practice as outlined below.

Influences of the organization

The degree to which lecturers can take the initiative in enhancing their teaching may depend as much on the nature of the organization they are working for, as their own interest and motivation. Teachers fairly new in post may find it particularly useful to assess their current teaching situation and to realize the importance of gaining the support of heads of departments in order for teaching initiatives to prove successful.

The overall plan

The centre should be a focussed facilitator of positive action to help formulate and implement a learning and teaching strategy for university-wide impact. It should be sensitive to the expectations and opportunities afforded by external agencies such as the Quality Assurance Authority (QAA). The centre should concentrate on forming functional links through secondment and collaboration to bring about actions with outcomes that make a difference. It should assure all parties that it is not attempting to duplicate or compete with existing activities or initiatives.

It should not be a central authority to pronounce on educational matters, giving out advice, or just giving out information, but provide resources to nurture self-development of staff so that they may become teaching authorities themselves.

It should hold a learning inventory of case studies where changes in teaching, ways of working with students and the uptake of new ideas are recorded. It should take responsibility for induction of new lecturers with teaching duties. The centre should organize meetings, conferences and forums that are largely participatory and publish a newsletter/journal and Web site. This can be achieved through leadership, organization and dedication of its staff and adequate funding.

Personnel positions, recognition and funding

Full-time members of staff would take a lead facilitatory role. Vital to the overall impact of the centre is the principle of collaboration. Two major ways in which this could be achieved would be through joint projects with other close functioning departments such as information services, and yearly secondment of staff from other academic departments. Staff throughout the university who make a longer-term commitment to the development of learning and teaching should be recognized, and a Teaching Fellowship scheme, critically evaluated over a period of five years, would help achieve this. Teachers who have shown outstanding educational development should be designated Teaching Champions and be funded to read a paper at an international educational conference.

Whilst the main impact of the centre should be on teachers who can cascade this influence to the learners, there is a good case for involving students at some stage to close the loop, to be assured that the educational developments facilitated by the centre are indeed enhancing students' learning. A promising initiative to produce this result would be to employ student liaison officers. These are experienced students who are willing to take a year out some way through their course (Bratley, Francis and Wilson, 2001). They could prove to be an invaluable resource. They will be in a position to help individual students find the support they need and thus may help student retention levels by keeping them on track. Student liaison officers will also be able to give important feedback to the centre that educational enhancements are having an appropriate impact.

A further evaluation of centre activities can be achieved through the appointment of dedicated Research Fellows, who can analyse the success of specific activities and overall functioning of the centre as a community. Central funding for full-time staff and students and Teaching and Research Fellowships and Teaching Champions would be necessary as these are completely new initiatives. However, some of the joint projects will promote shared responsibility between departments and the secondments should expand the educational teaching and research capacity of individuals within those departments. Some form of top-sliced funding to the centre may ensure that educational development occurs in departments appropriate to their needs, and joint projects with the centre would have a focus on functional outcomes.

Leadership of teaching

The institution can make statements of visions and values and institute manuals of policies and procedures, but unless deans and heads of departments support these, they will have limited impact (Candy, 1996). From questionnaires and semi-structured interviews with heads of academic departments, Martin *et al* (1997), were able to describe six categories of conceptions of leadership. The most inspired leadership to further progressive teaching in the widest educational context was described as having an emphasis on students' experience and initiating discussion with teachers and students on how to enable further improvement of this experience: a continuous curriculum change model.

The leader of the centre would clearly have to support this approach and be in a position to encourage other heads of departments. Martin *et al* (1997) categorized a further three types of fairly enlightened leadership that was willing to discuss with other teachers the students' experience, their roles, responsibilities, practice of teaching or the subjects and the discipline. Least enlightened concepts of leadership were where roles, responsibilities and teaching practices were imposed, or where structure and organization was imposed. Good academic leadership enables people to achieve and focusses on change whilst understanding the internal and external pressures on the educational process to achieve appropriate outcomes (Ramsden, 1998). The role of staff in the department must be to encourage and support their leader in accepting change and taking the necessary risks to develop more successful and satisfying learning and teaching.

Who should be a member of the centre? Monthly forum meetings should be open to all. A faculty-wide interprofessional education day for first-year students, in their first week, requires large numbers of staff to act as tutors for break-out groups – and this is an opportunity for staff to contribute and gain experience of interprofessional education in action.

Projects and collaborations

The centre will provide the public face of educational development for the institution. The centre can respond to specific issues and collaborate with other departments as task and finish exercises. An example could be a perceived difficulty of downloading and uploading materials to the MDV Web site. A collaborative exercise with the IT department could help clarify the primary educational issues on the one hand and the advantages and limitations of the software and hardware on the other. In these collaborative projects the primary aim is action to produce an achievable outcome. Action learning sets could be particularly helpful for participants to balancing reflection with action. Other collaborations could be considered long term, such as the establishment of a course and Postgraduate Certificate in Educational Development (PGCED) examination jointly with an existing awarding postgraduate section or department. The focussed inventory of educational development case studies could be catalogued and supported in a joint library services venture. Some important issues cross all disciplines and sections of society, such as communication, promotion of a healthy lifestyle, smoking cessation and coping with change. The centre should play an active role in brokering partnerships to further community.

The programme for the secondees

- There should be dedicated time for individual teachers to reflect on their current teaching position, to upgrade and update andragogy by following a set of core learning objective and values and the option of gaining a Postgraduate Certificate in Educational Development (PGCED);
- They should help to determine the learning and teaching needs in their own department;
- They should select an aspect of learning and teaching in their own department and institute educational change and write this up as a short case study;
- Paired with a cross-professional/disciplinary colleague they should contribute to a range of chosen and allocated activities within the centre;
- They should help with the peer assessment of teaching within their department;
- At the end of their appointments they should mentor the following secondees from their department.

Teaching Fellows and Champions

Two underlying threads of activity can be served by the creation of Teaching Fellows and Teaching Champions. Firstly, staff can be given recognition for educational development efforts that they are making and maintain a high profile public face for the centre. Secondly, they serve as levers to encourage excellence in teaching and provide encouragement for academics to choose a teaching career. Teaching Champions could be nominated sequentially during each year for recognition of work done in educational development. These could be awarded to secondees or others who have developed a presentation to be given at an international conference. A number of teachers who are willing to take on a project over a period of five years and are developing a track record in educational development could be awarded Teaching Fellowships. These could be established educators and those who have been secondees for one year and who would like to continue with their work. Teaching Fellows should:

- present an outline proposal for an educational project of five years' duration;
- make yearly interim reports on the progress made with their continuing professional development and contribution to the centre;

- with a cross-professional/disciplinary peer, act as advisor to the centre on an agreed topic;
- conduct a mentor role to secondees;
- contribute to the induction of lecturers with teaching duties;
- contribute to the functioning of the centre as negotiated.

Student liaison officers

Student liaison officers bridge the gap between students and the support and teaching they are offered. They do not offer advice themselves, but help students choose from the help options available. In some cases this could be for student support services. In others, it may be possible to help with academic problems. The approach in this role must be one of enthusiasm and impartiality. They should work in teams under the direction of a full-time member of staff at the centre. Student liaison officers should:

- attend an induction-training course on the structures of the university, educational development and roles of liaison officers;
- take a presentation role at the induction of the first-year students;
- direct students to sources of help;
- draw on the resources of the team of student liaison officers and leader full-time members of staff;
- attend secondary schools taking part in a widening access scheme;
- provide help for international and Erasmus exchange students;
- provide a student perspective at the learning and teaching forums;
- provide a student perspective at staff inductions.

Research Fellows

The proposal for a centre for educational development primarily involves lecturers who have a strong commitment to teaching. By their collaborative efforts the centre should help them realize their teaching potential and keep them teaching well and better. There is provision for programmes to enhance progressive development over a period of some years and a substantive feedback loop from students is proposed in the form of student liaison officers. The most powerful indicator for the success of the centre for educational development in an MDV setting is that interventions it facilitates should produce an appropriate healthcare outcome change (Kirkpatrick, 1967). Objective evidence from studies of the centre's early achievements and possible failures will be essential to plan ahead. There is, therefore, a fundamental need for at least a small body of researchers dedicated to the study of the centre and its community. A comparative study of exemplar teaching by Teaching Fellows using powerful healthcare indicators for success would be particularly demanding but may provide a base of evidence upon which to make further funding decisions. In addition, a qualitative study of the structure and function of the centre as a community may give important indicators for appropriate adjustment of sizing and remit of the centre at a review after a period of four or five years.

Alternative solutions

There is, sometimes, a temptation to muddle these learning and teaching enhancement approaches with management quality control that attempts to show that teaching standards are being monitored and improved. In some ways, this is a paper chase exercise that ensures that procedures are in place. It can be especially useful to get colleges to look again at what they are doing, expand provision when deficient, and attempt to equilibrate standards across disciplines. Management control systems, however enlightened, rarely blend well with concepts of teaching enhancement, which concentrate on the development of the individual teachers to respond to the learning needs of their students.

Learning in MDV education must be object- or context-specific so cannot but have a vested professional interest, but what seems important is the realization of interdependence in the health professions. Many different professions are needed for the overall care of the health needs of the population and of patients. Further, we should respect the qualities of these other professionals and understand the limitations of our own competence. Also, we have common ground in our links with ethical issues of diversity, inclusiveness and connectedness. In essence, this means that we need to promote community, in which we appreciate and recognize our differences and similarities.

Should the centre have professional advisers who can take on some of the teaching role of academics? One feature of the new universities is the development of those in the registry or the faculty administration who have an academic advisory function (Guest, 2001). Ensuring students present modules on time and organizing course changes and pastoral care, are taken on by these advisers. Does this enhance the learning experience of students? A one-stop shop for students' generic needs, such as finance, housing, writing and basic IT skill development and student counselling is appealing, as students are likely to find the help they want when they need it. However, this system may distance the students more from their teachers, who will spend less time with them. The academics will be released to spend more time on their research! In most circumstances this is hardly a means to enhance teaching. Advisory function officers may have a useful registry role especially in the running of complex MDV courses.

Services and support

The basic human needs must be satisfied before learning can take place, and those who provide counselling provide a service to help students with their domestic situations or generic learning difficulties so that they have a mind to deal with their specific subject learning and professional development. Counselling must be, and must be seen to be, confidential and a low-key peripheral activity. It would not gain from being brought into a central place except to advertise the fact that it is available and so permit ready uptake.

Should the centre be virtual?

Virtual learning environments (VLEs) are available as resources both for students and teachers to learn specific skills or knowledge. Distance virtual learning obviously has the advantage of availability at any time with a simple computer connection, does not eat into dedicated time, is available to all and can be accompanied by an assessment and even a certificate to warrant that learning has taken place (eg, TRIP Database, 2002). However, VLE programmes cannot encompass a great deal of variation, do not open up networks of communication and do not directly further community activity across professions. The centre could be linked to virtual learning environments or become linked to a managed learning environment (MLE). A computer network system that works consistently and provides means of access to quality information quickly and permits communication between teachers and students must be an essential resource for a centre to enhance learning and teaching, but the physical structure and facility does not in itself provide insight into what actions to take nor what motivates a community towards teaching enhancement.

Is a learning and teaching centre an educational research establishment?

Teachers who are trying to enhance their practice will be constantly asking themselves, 'How can we do better?' They will be planning and taking action to achieve that. This kind of educational action research occurs when teachers aim to improve their teaching at the grass roots level by incorporating the views and expressions of the stakeholders of the process, be they students or patients. Thinking behind the research takes them through the Kolb learning cycle (see Chapter 4) of reflecting on their teaching, planning changes and improvements, acting on these and observing the outcomes with both researcher and researched contributing to the overall findings. This kind of research must be part and parcel of enhancing learning and teaching. Educational research using psychometric tests or phenomenography is often carried out by researchers on other teachers and their students. The irony is that the complexity of formulating the research questions, filling in grant applications, the data collection and interpretation of results and preparation for publication pull the researcher away from teaching itself, so that generally researchers do not directly enhance their own teaching.

A constructive way forward may be collaboration between researchers and teachers. The major function of the personnel at the learning and teaching centre may be to act as intermediary or broker between the teachers who would like to improve their teaching but do not have research experience, and the researchers who would like to work with valid teaching materials. The centre should also create other opportunities for teachers to step outside of their teaching duties for a year or so and facilitate research for a time. The community approach may also permit cross-professional research. A self-development approach will realize the potential of individuals at different times in their professional lives.

Should the centre take on the whole of professional development?

Academics carry out many management roles and need training. Much of this is not directly related to teaching although there may be some spill over. There seems little point in competing with the Personnel or Human Resources Department to provide management training. The centre could lose the focus of educational development. However, there may be scope for collaboration on joint issues such as coping with change, communication and motivation.

Taking teaching seriously

Those lecturers who have volunteered to be secondees at the centre will be taking their teaching seriously, following the literature and seeing how they can develop their approach to facilitating the learning of their students. Saroyan and Amundsen (2001) say that a change in practice occurs when teachers change their basic assumptions held about themselves as learners, their role and the goal of education and that reflection is the key to the process. They propose a new model of teaching for higher education that contains four elements: conceptions, knowledge, action and context. They suggest that conceptions, which are defined as one's beliefs about learning and teaching, determine the kind of knowledge one draws upon to complete the educational task. Knowledge includes the subject matter as well as knowledge of pedagogy/andragogy related to the subject, task and learners. Action is the enactment of the teaching task, which occurs in the overall educational context.

The characteristics of good teaching are, broadly, that it is student-centred, so teaching is a form of facilitating learning but where clear objectives are stated.

Good teaching, they claim, occurs when teachers are able to act out their thoughts and bring reflection into the process; ie, when there is convergence between conceptions and actions. They make the point that to gain feedback from the students is an enlightened approach as far as it goes, but far more is needed to evaluate teaching in this wider context. Apart from questionnaires they suggest studies of free writing and journal-keeping, records of critical incidents, needs assessment, a teacher behaviour inventory and the use of metaphor to build a greater picture of how the teacher helps generate a suitable educational climate for the student to facilitate learning.

If the programme for secondees is based on this kind of approach, the individual will be able to carry out some of these reflective activities, but will be encouraged to work collaboratively with a cross-professional/disciplinary peer to help enhance each other's teaching. The reflective practice based on action learning sets of a small group of, say six, secondees will help participants to focus on their individual actions, how they give peer support and how they can contribute to the activities of the centre.

The personal side of learning and teaching

[We want] 'to make citizens and workers but also we ultimately want to make human beings who will live life to the fullest' (Dewey, 1916). The influence of the teacher should not be underestimated. Candy, Crebert and O'Leary (1994) found that the behaviour of academic staff was more influential in determining student attitudes towards learning throughout their lives than information given in official documents with institutional rhetoric. It is therefore appropriate for the secondee to analyse where they are placed in their career, and in their understanding and commitment to learning and teaching. The opportunities for teachers to express themselves may vary in a number of ways. Boyer (1989) brought in the concept that academic life may express itself in the form of seasons, wherein some teaching, research or administration may be the major focus of attention. Even within the field of teaching, there may be a specific focus of activity, say of developing curricular structures or content, using various teaching methods, involvement in the assessment methods and examinations or taking on an academic support role. The secondee is encouraged to follow a core curriculum of current educational concepts that may enable personal and institutional change and development:

- The first fundamental concept is the central one of understanding how students learn. This includes psychology of the predilection of some students to certain styles of learning and the characteristics of a good learner (see Chapters 7, 11 and 12). The current concepts of the importance of a deep approach to learning and constructive alignment of teacher with the student and the use of learning contracts are covered (Biggs, 1999; Anderson, Boud and Sampson, 1996).

- A second concept is the value of evidence-based practice in the clinic and the classroom (Sackett *et al*, 2000; Belfield *et al*, 2001).
- A third concept is the aspiration to ensure that MDV education is patient-centred and that, in the early stages of training in particular, there is provision of appropriate clinical simulation (Hasle, 1994: Chapter 13).
- A fourth concept is that of individual ethical behaviour within the professional and interprofessional context (Crawford, 2001).

Conclusion

The opportunities for educational development in MDV have never been greater for the individual lecturer. However, with a centre that can focus collaborative activities between enthusiastic educators from these professions and beyond, the scope of activities increases manifoldly. The temptation to make the centre an all-inclusive part of registry is resisted, although it is argued that it should be highly collaborative with other departments and service sections of the university. The focus should be clearly on the enhancement of learning and teaching. Demarcated roles for various members of staff and students are suggested. A leader with vision but one who is willing to adopt a continuous change model for the curriculum is advocated. The major organizational method to ensure the centre has direct relevance to everyday teaching in the departments is through secondment of lecturers into the centre and their continuing work and return to the departments. Creation of Teaching Fellowships helps provide an optional longer-term strand of further progression and development for some of these staff. Employment of student liaison officers shows a commitment to and a functional means of ensuring feedback on the student experience. Research Fellows dedicated to studying the centre as a working community, and as a means of enhancing teaching and healthcare outcomes will provide objective data that can be used to plan the centre's future development.

References

Anderson, G, Boud, D and Sampson, J (1996) *Learning Contracts: A practical guide*, Kogan Page, London

Belfield, C *et al* (2001) Measuring effectiveness for best evidence medical education: a discussion, *Medical Teacher*, **23** (2), pp 164–70

Biggs, J (1999) *Teaching for quality learning at university: What the student does*, SRHE and OUP, Buckingham

Boyer, E L (1989) Connectedness Through Liberal Education, in *Curriculum Planning: A New Approach*, eds G Hass and F W Parkay, 6th edn, pp 525–31, Allyn and Bacon, Boston

Bratley, S, Francis, P and Wilson, L (2001) *Bridging the Gap*, presented at First Annual Conference on Academic Advising, Luton University, 11–12 July

Candy, P C, Crebert, R G and O'Leary, J (1994) Developing lifelong learners through undergraduate education, *National Board of Employment, Education and Training Commissioned Report*, **28**, Australian Government Publishing Service, Canberra

Candy, P (1996) Promoting Lifelong Learning: Academic Developers and the University as a Learning Organization, *International Journal for Academic Development*, **1**, pp 7–18

Coventry University (2002) *Centre for Higher Educational Development* [Online] http://www.ched.coventry.ac.uk/ched/aboutched/index.htm

Crawford, P D (2001) Educating for Moral Ability: reflections on moral development based on Vygotsky's theory of concept formation, *Journal of Moral Education*, **30** (2), pp 113–29

Dewey, J (1916) *Democracy and Education*, MacMillan, New York

Fry, H, Ketteridge, S and Marshall, S (1999) *A Handbook for Teaching and Learning in Higher Education: Enhancing Academic Practice*, Kogan Page, London

Genn, J M (2001) AMEE Medical Education Guide No 23 (Part 1): Curriculum, environment, climate, quality and change in medical education – a unifying perspective, *Medical Teacher*, **23**, pp 337–44

Gibbs, G, Habeshaw, S and Habeshaw, T (1988) *53 Interesting Ways to Appraise Your Teaching*, 1997 reprint edn, *TES*/University of Exeter, Exeter

Guest, K (2001) *Enhancing the Academic Advisory Function in Higher Education*, Keynote Speech, First Annual Conference, Luton, July

Hasle, J L (1994) Analysis of the Costs and Benefits of Using Standardized Patients to Help Teach Physical Diagnosis, *Academic Medicine*, **69** (7), pp 567–70

Kirkpatrick, D I (1967) Evaluation of Training, in *Training and Development Handbook*, eds R Craig and I Mittel, McGraw-Hill, New York

Martin, E *et al* (1997) Heads' of academic departments conceptions of leadership of teaching, in *Improving Student Learning Through Course Design*, eds C Rust and G Gibbs, pp 356–61, OUP, Oxford

Race, P (1999) *2000 Tips for Lecturers*, Kogan Page, London

Ramsden, P (1998) *Learning to Lead in Higher Education*, Routledge, London

Randall, F and Downie, R S (1999) *Palliative Care Ethics: A Companion for all Specialties*, 2nd edn, OUP, Oxford

Sackett, D L *et al* (2000) *Evidence-based Medicine: How to Practice and Teach EBM*, 2nd edn, Churchill Livingston, Edinburgh

Saroyan, A and Amundsen, C (2001) Evaluating University Teaching: time to take stock, *Assessment and Evaluation in Higher Education*, **26** (4), pp 341–53

TRIP Database (2002) *TRIP Database* [Online] http://www.tripdatabase.com/vlc/

2

Culture, collegiality and collaborative learning

George Brown, Madeleine Rohlin and Michael Manogue

Introduction

The relationship between culture, collegiality and collaborative learning may appear to be a conundrum to many readers. In this chapter we unravel the conundrum and show its importance for the education of MDV students in this, the 21st century. At its heart is the question: how should MDV students be prepared for a newly emerging society whose structure and form is uncertain? To answer that question, one needs to explore the changes in society, the cultures of MDV Schools and their positive and negative effects upon collegiality and the effects of collegiality upon learning. To complicate matters further, the relationships between culture, collegiality and learning are not unidirectional. Changes in any one of these may have consequential changes in the others. Clearly there can be no simple answer to this question. Rather one can only offer perspectives for readers to consider and reflect upon. The issues are deep.

What goes on in learning is shaped by the strength of collegiality, which in its turn is shaped by MDV culture. This culture is susceptible to changes in society. We say susceptible because there is often a cultural lag between what occurs in MDV Schools and what may be appropriate in a changing society. Despite the exhortations of various official reports such as the GMC (1993) the GDC (1997) and the Lucke report (RCVS, 1991), there have not yet been radical changes in MDV education in Britain nor in medical or dental education in the United States (Enarson and Burg, 1992; Field, 1995).

Moving towards a learning society?

There is no doubt that advanced societies are changing rapidly and more rapidly than less developed societies. This widening gap has implications for healthcare systems and MDV education in different parts of the world. The e-revolution has brought in its wake global communications and markets and consequent shifts in developed countries away from an 'industrial' society. Broadly speaking there are two views of these changes in post-industrial societies. The first is pessimistic: a closed society is emerging. The second is optimistic: a learning society is emerging.

The darker view is that the core values of the industrial society will penetrate more deeply into companies, educational organizations and individuals. Increasing bureaucratization, in the form of complex detailed procedures, will permeate healthcare systems and MDV education. Codes of practice, manuals of quality assurance and programme specifications will limit the freedom of MDVs, MDV teachers and MDV students. De-skilling, perhaps proletariatization of professional groups will occur (Halsey, 1992). Large private international companies will strengthen further their grip on research agendas, the healthcare provided and perhaps the curriculum. The drive for profits will lead to short-term contracts for organizations and individuals. Control and conformity will be the agenda, not freedom to learn.

The optimistic view is shown in Table 2.1. The changes that will occur are qualitative rather than quantitative. In a 'learning society' the stance towards resources, human beings, education and leadership will be different compared to those of the 'industrial society'. There will be a focus on human beings and their development of knowledge and learning both as individuals and as members of teams or of organizations. The tasks will no longer be merely standardized routines but they will be continuously redefined and they will demand new patterns of thinking. As individuals we will have to be 'proactive'. Leadership will not be implemented via control systems but by shared visions and values. In the learning society, organizations/institutions will be challenged to develop capabilities for learning and change, to become 'learning organizations'. This definition implies an approach where the culture within the organization encourages learning and development as a continuous and conscious process, which is shared amongst all members. Collaborative learning is vital because teams, not individuals are the learning unit in contemporary organizations. Besides, collaborative learning, a learning organization benefits from mental models, the building of shared visions and personal mastery (Senge, 1992). We do not know which of these images of the future will prevail but we do know that if we are to help MDV students to learn, we must work with them for the future rather than train them for the immediate present.

Table 2.1 The industrial society and the learning society – a comparison

	Industrial Society	Learning Society
most important resources	capital	knowledge
raw	resources	time
most important foundation	investments	learning
driving force	accumulation of money	accumulation of knowledge
power base	control of money	control of knowledge
principles for leadership	with control systems	with values
economic key figures	visions	missions
key words	control	trust

MDV culture

Every MDV practitioner is familiar with the notion of culture as a medium in which organisms flourish, reproduce, survive or perish. The organisms interact with the culture, and in so doing may change the culture. In social sciences, this notion of culture is extended to include the culture of a society, an organization, a group or an individual. At the societal level, culture embraces the technologies, artefacts, religions, the arts, core values, beliefs and myths of a society. At the organizational and group level, culture usually refers to the artefacts, shared values, attitudes, expectations and patterns of behaviour. Sometimes this form of culture is referred to as ethos, climate, learning context, learning environment or simply environment (Genn, 2001). At the level of the individual, culture refers to the internalized values, attitudes and consequent behaviours, which occur through the processes of socialization (sometimes described as enculturation or acculturation).

The analysis of culture may seem remote from the everyday practices of MDV but one should be wary of dismissing it as irrelevant. For example, the values of North American culture and North European culture are different and lead to very different healthcare systems and different emphases in MDV education. The culture of MDV Schools may include collegiality and the culture of collegiality may include collaborative learning. The culture of an MDV School can affect the morale, mode of working, and achievements of its staff and students. The culture of a group within a school or hospital can shape the attitudes and values of its participants (Wilson and Pirrie, 1999).

Subcultures within a culture have some things in common with all other subcultures in that culture, some things in common with some others, and some characteristics that are specific to that subculture. The commonalities are more like family resemblances than clear-cut categories. For example, the cultures of Medical, Dental and Veterinary Schools differ and differ amongst themselves; groups of orthopaedic surgeons tend to have different attitudes and values from groups of paediatricians yet all are medical graduates. Vets who work with large animals are somewhat different from vets who work with small animals. Prosthetic dentists and oral radiologists differ in some attitudes. These differences are partly attributable to self-selection for membership of the subculture, the mode of working in the speciality and the subculture itself.

Finally it is worth considering what methods of studying cultural differences are available. We do not yet have precise methods of delineating different learning cultures but there are some pointers. We do know from the work of Entwistle and Ramsden (1983) and Entwistle and Tait (1990) that students' approaches to learning are associated with a set of characteristics of a learning environment. The findings indicate that departments where 'good' teaching was reported were strongly oriented towards deep learning. Good teaching included such variables as openness, accessibility of staff, help with specific difficulties and perceived freedom to learn. Poor teaching included such variables as ineffective lecturing, heavy workloads, inappropriate assessment and lack of freedom to learn. In these departments the orientation towards reproductive learning was strong. The subsequent Course Experience Questionnaire of Ramsden (1992) and his studies of leadership (Ramsden, 1998) provide further clues. There are the beginnings of promising developments from the seminal work of Becher (Becher and Trowler, 2001) on cultures of disciplines. The ethnographic approaches being used by Gentle (2001) are promising ways of deepening understanding of cultures. Extensions of the DREEM (Dundee Ready Education Environment Measure) measures and of Harden's model for evaluating educational developments might also yield interesting insights (Harden, Sowden and Dunn, 1984).

Commonalities of MDV culture

Despite the subcultural differences of MDV culture, it has at least three current commonalties: repair, healing and care; scientific positivism and a mode of education based largely on transmission and imitation.

Repair, healing and care

Repair, healing and care are likely to remain a commonality although the nature of repair and healing is changing and the social dimension of care is becoming increasingly important in some healthcare systems. This dimension includes palliative care, care of the elderly, drug addiction and the impact of the bio-social environment on nutrition. Rather more than drugs are needed to tackle these problems. An additional dimension of lifestyle is likely to become more prevalent. This ranges from aesthetic demands of patients or their clients to selection of the sex of offspring. These changes have long-term ethical and educational implications for MDV curricula.

Positivism and humanism in MDV culture and education

This is perhaps the most important feature of MDV culture and therefore of MDV Schools. The underlying argument of this section may be expressed, perhaps too simply, in a syllogistic form:

- Research drives an MDV School's values, its culture, its medical education, its curriculum teaching, learning and assessment.
- The research methods are almost wholly scientific.
- Therefore the culture, MDV education and its curriculum, teaching, learning and assessment methods are almost wholly scientific.
- Therefore humanistic approaches to students and patients are undervalued.

There is a tension in existing MDV culture between the need for 'scientific rigour' in the treatment of disease and the needs of patients and communities (see Table 2.2), although the slightly different pole of 'whole animal' rather than 'person' is required for veterinary medicine. The tension has been in the culture since at least the 16th century (O'Malley, 1970). At the beginning of the century the quality of doctors was thought to have been at risk because of their lack of 'scientific rigour'. At the beginning of the 21st century there is a swing towards the needs of the community and the patient. To quote Jolly (1998: 122): 'we need again to appraise what educational activities are beneficial and or feasible within the developing healthcare systems'. Given the recent reports on errors in patient care (Kohn, Corrigan and Donaldson, 1999; Vincent *et al*, 2001), this concern is all the more pressing.

Table 2.2 Contrasting views in MDV culture

The Body	The Person
treating the disease the patient has	treating the patient who has the disease
the site of biomedical knowledge	understanding the person in their context
clinical, disease-related realities	the patient's life world
clinical competence	caring competence
technical skills and knowledge	social skills and respect for persons

This tension within MDV culture has its roots in two contrasting ideologies (sets of cultural values), which emerged strongly in the 19th century. These have been labelled *erklarung*, or scientific explanation, and *verstehen*, the search for personal meaning and understanding (Ricoeur, 1981; Brown and Atkins, 1988). Table 2.3 shows the contrasting poles of these ideologies.

Table 2.3 Contrasting poles of scientific positivism and humanism

Erklarung:	**Verstehen:**
the search for scientific explanations, 'truths' about the real world	the search for meaning and understanding of the persons and life worlds
scientific	humanistic
experimentally based	interpretative
objective	intersubjective
hypothesis-driven	hypothesis-emergent
quantitative	qualitative
measurement	judgement
statistical reliability	linguistic consistency
statistical validity	consensual validity
detachment	involvement
controlled environment	open environment

Positivism has been, and is, the predominant force in MDV culture. It is encapsulated in Galileo's phrase 'Measure that which is measurable, make measurable that which is not'. Scientific advances have led to increased life expectancy and improved quality of life, particularly in developed countries, but satisfaction of MDV professionals and patients may be declining whilst health costs rise (Le Fanu, 1999). A few of the advances have benefited only a small minority who can afford expensive treatments and almost all the advances have benefited large pharmaceutical and bio-technological companies. What has been neglected in this enterprise is the care of patients as human beings. But since there is little profit to be gained, the research and development of this aspect of care has been underfunded.

The drive for scientific research has permeated the culture of MDV Schools. Tenure, promotion and status are largely dependent on scientific research and on obtaining research grants. Research into MDV education has also been dominated by this paradigm. In a survey of research in medical education carried out between 1976 and 1996, Dimitroff and Davies (1996) found that of 3,900 articles, most studies were scientifically based and largely concerned with the effects of a particular teaching method. There was no research reported in medical journals on the socialization process, few qualitative-based articles and even fewer on Medical Schools and hospitals as social institutions. Such research is published usually in Social Science journals and texts (Becker *et al*, 1961; Atkinson, 1977; Arluke, 1980; Sinclair, 1998). An exception to this rule is a recent article by Maheux *et al* (2000) who surveyed the perceptions of students and junior physicians of their senior physicians as humanistic teachers and doctors (response rate of 69 per cent of 1,039). Forty per cent of the senior clerks thought their physicians were not good role models as doctors or teachers. More than half thought that their teachers did not value human contact with them. There was however a highly significant difference in views between those taught by problem-based learning (PBL) in innovative schools and those taught in traditional schools. PBL and innovative schools, it seems, may have a more humanistic culture.

Recently there have been attempts to 'humanize' MDV education. Courses in ethics, literature and studies of cultural values are now more commonplace. Palliative education may be beginning to have an impact. But these courses take place in a culture and research orientation that is predominantly positivistic. Chance conditioning, attitudes of MDV teachers and the hidden curriculum are likely to be more influential than short courses, particularly if those courses are perceived by deans, MDV teachers and students as marginal to MDV practice. Cribb and Bignold (1999) have argued that until the research culture of Medical Schools contains a strong humanistic component there are unlikely to be changes at the level of teaching. What is required is a collegial approach based on collaborative learning, an approach that ensures scientific rigour but is permeated by humanistic values.

Transmission and imitation

Transmission and imitation have been the predominant modes of education in MDV Schools for centuries. Medical education consisted largely of lectures followed by an apprenticeship with a master. The students learnt largely through rote, they were tested by methods of recall and then allowed to learn to practice. Learning to practice was done through modelling the master by observing, listening and copying. Clinical teaching consisted of 'looking over the shoulder' of the apprentice at work. Elements of this approach are still with us today, but by the beginning of the 20th century most Medical Schools had incorporated the notion of medicine as science and later, similar trends were found in Dental and Veterinary Schools. All MDV Schools shared these characteristics:

- a basic science course followed by clinical sciences;
- teachers as experts and authorities;
- clinical experience is provided in different settings.

In the latter stages of the 20th century this approach was beginning to appear anachronistic. Various reports have advocated the use of integrated approaches along the lines of clinical problem-solving, an emphasis upon community-based experience and patient care in a diverse society (O'Neill, 1992; RCVS, 1991; GMC, 1993; GDC, 1997). Some MDV Schools have, or are changing their curriculum, although in the United Kingdom they are hampered by the strait-jacket imposed by the QAA (Quality Assurance Agency) (2001). The notion of the teacher as universal expert is no longer as tenable in an age when knowledge is increasing exponentially. The new emphasis is upon the development of an autonomous, self-directed, reflective learner. Clinical experience has been shown to be variable and often unrelated to the basic sciences. Jolly (1998) likens clinical experience to minestrone soup, prepared by different chefs rather than carefully planned educational experiences. All of these point to the renewed importance of collegiality and collaborative learning: 'When education narrows its scope of inquiry, it reduces a culture's power to adapt to change' (Bruner, 1996: 15).

Neglected aspects of MDV education

Beneath transmission and imitation are lurking deeper neglected issues that affect the way young adults become young MDV professionals. For it is not only knowledge that is transmitted and professionalism that is imitated, culture in its wider sense of shared values is transmitted and other aspects of behaviour, sometimes non-professional ones, are role-modelled. This hidden curriculum is, arguably, at least as important in the socialization of MDV students. The neglect of studies and considerations of these issues is largely because they do not fit the scientific paradigm and, perhaps, because they confront MDV Schools with problems that they do not wish to face. Cribb and Bignold (1999) take up these arguments in their stimulating article on the reflexive (reflective) Medical School. They point to the loss of idealism among medical students, the demands of survival, the problem of side-tracking, learning to work with bodies, the rituals of attainment and the issue of professional identity. All of these might be termed 'emotional socialization'. They suggest that the changing gender and ethnic composition of student cohorts may have an effect upon the culture of Medical Schools. In addition, one can point to cognitive loss, the decline of deep learning in conventional undergraduate courses (see below and Coles, 1998).

Both emotional socialization and cognitive loss in MDV education contain tensions. One needs to teach, in a profound sense, 'detached concern' so that students can cope with aggressive treatments of bodies whilst respecting patients as persons. Until recently, firms had a role to play here and collaborative learning and mentoring continue to have a role. Cognitive loss is primarily a product of the overloaded curriculum and its assessment (Ramsden, 1992). Perhaps it is time to ponder again the words of a distinguished educator, Lawrence Stenhouse (1975), who said that we must stop thinking of the curriculum as a fixed race course and begin to think of it as a tool for stimulating and directing active learning: we must be attempting something worthwhile as well as achieving what it attempts.

Collegiality

Collegiality has been described as 'a necessary compromise between "I" and "they" to make "we" in every sphere of life' (Handy, 1995). The term like its sister terms 'college' and 'colleagues' springs from the verb *collegere*: to read together. Gradually the term collegiality has come to mean working together as equals, the sharing of decisions and the joint exploration of evidence, meanings and values. Sometimes the term collegiality with its implications of empowerment, sharing and working together, is contrasted with the term bureaucracy, which emphasizes role allocation in a hierarchy, supervision, management and accountability. Herein lie conflicts. In higher education management there is a drive away from collegiality towards bureaucracy (Kogan, Moses and El-Khawas, 1994). In learning in higher education there is a tentative drive towards collegiality. At the systemic level, the conflict is manifest in the complex specifications of Academic Review (QAA, 2001), which imply that students should have little say in determining the intended outcomes of their learning and the Institute of Learning and Teaching (ILT, 1999) which, in its statement of professional values, stresses: 'respect for individual learners and for their development and empowerment' and 'commitment to the development of learning communities, including students, teachers and all those engaged in learning support'. These conflicts are felt in some MDV Schools in the conflicts between the administrative demands for quality assurance procedures and the desire to focus on the practicalities of providing effective learning environments.

Strands of collegiality

There are three strands of collegiality that merit consideration: relations between staff, relations between staff and students and the school as a learning organization.

Relationships between staff and between staff and students

Good relationships between staff are not only important for them and the health of the organization; they also provide role models for future generations of MDV students. Good collegial relationships does not mean there should be no debate or controversy between colleagues but rather that they work in a cultural ethos that encourages active open debate among equals.

This notion should be extended to the relationship between staff and students. Students of today have to adapt to a society that will change more rapidly than the society that many of us grew up in. Even if they do not change specialities, their specialities will change. So to equip them for their roles as professionals one has to empower them so they become independent, reflective learners who want to continue to learn long after they have graduated. This approach may require major shifts in the minds of some MDV teachers. The concepts of teaching and learning, as expressed in course documents, are not always matched by the concepts used in practice. Underpinning many of the learning and assessment tasks is often the notion of learning as reproduction of knowledge rather the search for understanding (Bowden and Marton, 1998) and the concept of teaching is primarily based on transmission rather the organization of learning (Trigwell, Prosser and Waterhouse, 1999). Similar gaps have been identified between the rhetoric and reality of assessment (Manogue, Brown and Foster, 2001). These changes are all the more difficult because they ask teachers to give up power, to change their role from expert teller of truths to a designer of learning environments in which students are guided, facilitated and challenged to seek knowledge and understanding for themselves.

MDV Schools as learning organizations

The concept of the learning organization has its origins in management theory whereas collegiality comes from an older, academic tradition. They share a common concern with values but they differ on the importance of common 'vision'. In a sense, all MDV Schools are learning organizations in that they organize with varying degrees of success, the learning of their students. But not all are learning organizations in the sense that management theorists such as Senge (1992) and Pedler, Burgoyne and Boydell (1997) use the term. For them, leadership is diffused through the organization and the vision and values of the organization are shared. They advocate that the approach of 'command and control' should be replaced by a culture whose core values include learning from the experiences and reflections of the members of the organizations, self-development opportunities, a learning climate and participant decision-making. For these to occur, Jones (1996) argues for the development of collaborative interpersonal skills such as listening, openness, self-reflection, respect for persons and tolerance. In her text she reviews the literature of change management and she suggests that the high failure rate in innovations is attributable to 'the neglect of core soft skills and the inability to convert from the traditional hierarchical "command and control" to a collaborative learning culture' (Jones, 1996: 13).

A key feature of learning organizations is the nature of leadership. The consensus seems to be that leadership should be based on the values of collaboration, trust, exemplary practice, shared values and inspiration. This form of leadership is sometimes described as 'transformation' leadership. Departments or schools in which transformation leadership was manifest in fair and firm management and there was recognition that the development of staff was a high priority 'were more likely to contain teachers who reported student focused approaches to teaching. They are also less likely to report teacher focused approaches... Moreover the students in these units rated the teaching more highly...' (Ramsden, 1998: 66).

We do not know of any work in MDV education that is comparable to Ramsden's studies. But our observations of many MDV Schools in Europe suggest that few warrant the technical label of 'learning organizations'. Nor is 'transformational leadership' evident in many schools or their departments. This may be because hierarchies of command resonate with hypothetic-deductive methods, with the earlier tradition of master apprenticeship and with the transmission-imitation model of teaching. Whatever the reasons, the emerging notion of MDV Schools as learning organizations is crucial for the development of culture, collegiality and collaborative learning in MDV education.

Collegiality: the foundations of lifelong learning

It is generally agreed that one of the primary aims of MDV education is to lay the foundations of lifelong learning (RCVS, 1991; GMC, 1993; GDC, 1997). Dewey enunciated this view in his writing on education: 'the most important attitude that can be formed is that of desire to go on learning' (Dewey, 1997: 48). The distinguished medical educator, Osler, observed at the beginning of the last century that: 'The hardest conviction to get into the mind of a beginner is that the education upon which he is engaged is not a college course, not a medical course, but a life course, for which the work of a few years under teachers is but a preparation'(Osler, 1914, cited by Jennett, 1993: 18).

The question is, what is the best foundation for lifelong learning in a culture that is changing rapidly and in which knowledge is exploding? The answer to the question lies in the approaches to learning that students adopt and these are shaped by their experiences of the curriculum and its hidden components. The themes of curriculum and learning is discussed in this book by Sweet and, inter alia, by Tomasello, Kruger and Ratner (1993), Biggs (1999), Brown, Bull and Pendlebury (1997) and Coles (1998). Broadly speaking, these reviews lead to the conclusion that students continue to learn best when:

- they actively search for understanding;
- they reflect upon their learning;
- they perceive the learning and assessment tasks as relevant to their intended career;
- they feel safe enough in their learning environment to take risks in their discussion and thinking;
- the objectives or learning outcomes are perceived as clear or meaningful;
- their emotional needs and social needs are satisfied through a sense of security and belonging to a supportive group.

Now look at the traditional curriculum that developed in the 20th century (see the previous section on transmission and imitation). We asked students to learn a vast array of knowledge in basic sciences, which at a much later date they are expected to apply in clinical situations that they have no experience or knowledge of! The objectives of the individual modules in basic sciences are often clear, but their links, in the students' minds, may not be clearly related to their intended career. The mode of teaching is largely lecture-based and the practicals are usually at the level of demonstration and recipe. The assessment load is burdensome and the mode of assessment often consists of brief responses to narrow questions – short answers and MCQs (multiple-choice questions). Given these characteristics of the curriculum it is hardly surprising that the students adapt learning strategies for surface learning. As Coles (1985) and Newble and Clarke (1996) in medical education and Biggs (1987) in higher education have shown, students often begin their courses with high scores on deep learning and low scores on surface learning. Within a year or so, they have high scores on surface learning and low scores on deep learning. Learning may be perceived as a 'trial by ordeal' based on memory tasks rather than a preparation for a career, based upon a search for understanding and meaning. This early socialization does not meet the criteria of how students learn best. It does not augur well for deep, meaningful, lifelong learning.

In contrast, a collegial approach fits the research evidence more closely. It involves treating students as junior colleagues, who through discourse, guided study and practice and self-directed learning are encouraged to actively search for meaning and relevant new knowledge. Evidence from innovative Medical Schools (Newble and Clarke, 1986; Schmidt and Molen, 2001) suggest that attitudes towards lifelong learning and continuing professional development is better by students from innovative Medical Schools. The message is clear. Collegiality is a better foundation for lifelong learning than didacticism.

Collaborative learning

If collegiality is the foundation of lifelong learning, then collaborative learning is the method of laying that foundation. In collaborative learning, tutors and students work together on common tasks. These include problem-based learning in its many forms, learning contracts, portfolios, team projects, joint assessment of practical tasks, case-based learning, student-based grand rounds and community-based education.

Collaborative learning is both a process through which people teach each other and themselves and a vehicle for teaching social and communication skills. Its values are manifold. It provides opportunities to develop and test thinking and practice, it provides support and motivation to learn, in enriches learning, it develops social and communication skills, and it provides a basis for team work – an increasingly important feature of MDV work with patients, colleagues and members of the wider healthcare team. Last but not least, it provides humanistic role models for students who, when they become professionals, may well change the socialization process of future MDV students.

However, it would be wrong to assume collaborative learning should be the only method of learning. There is nothing wrong with experts talking with novices. Lectures and occasional overviews have their place providing they do not usurp the development of active learning. Individual practice of diagnostic and other practical skills is necessary although these can be practised in a collaborative context. Self-directed learning and thinking is at least as important as collaborative learning. Indeed collaborative learning can be conceived of as a medium for developing autonomous learning, a halfway house between teacher dependants and professional autonomy.

Competence and collaborative learning

Competence is often regarded as the ability to perform to an acceptable standard in a given context. Performativity is its cardinal feature. Such a view is useful but narrow. It leads to highly detailed analysis and assessments of the here and now. If one is preparing students for their future careers one needs to go beyond this form of confidence to help students cope with unknown situations. As Bowden and Marton (1998: 6) observe, '... [we] are supposed to prepare students for handling situations in the future. These future situations are more or less unknown... We have to prepare the students for the unknown by means of the known...' The issue here is, apparently, one of transferability. Transfer, in so far as it is achievable, is most likely to occur when a learner understands the key principles and the context in which the principles are to be applied. To achieve this goal we need to provide students with a rich variety of learning tasks derived from different contexts so they become adept at recognizing similarities and difference of context, they come to learn in which context which principles apply and do not apply. They need to consider holistically the ethical and psychological issues, costs and possible unintended consequences of their actions. Reflection and collaborative learning can aid this form of competence far better than a regime of transmission and imitation.

Problem-solving, critical thinking and creativity

Critical and creative thinking is the bedrock of problem-solving and problem-solving is the basis of learning for the future. If you want students to be better problem-solvers, to think critically or to think creatively then you need to provide the conditions in which these capabilities can flourish. We know from studies of small groups and small group teaching (see Chapter 5 by Joy Crosby; Brown and Atkins, 1988 and Jacques, 2000) that the optimal conditions for the formation of attitudes and the development of these capabilities are ownership of the problem or task; a safe learning environment in which participants can take risks, mutual respect amongst members of the group yet a willingness to change ideas and a facilitator who asks probing, reflective questions. In the early life of a group, the facilitator may be a tutor; through explicit modelling and reflective discussion the role of the facilitator can be taken over by other members of the group.

This approach has all the features of collegiality and collaborative learning fulfils these optimal conditions. Even tutorials based on learning contracts can be a context in which the tutor's role becomes relatively minor: the student asks the right questions and offers the answers. Common dangers that inhibit the growth of these capabilities are that the leader is authoritarian, asks quick-fire recall questions rather than thought questions, does not encourage student–student interaction, and does not move discussion on from description of events or facts to the search for reasons and causes (Brown, Bull and Pendlebury, 1997).

Communicative competence and collaborative learning

There is a growing awareness in the importance of communication between professionals and clients. Studies indicate that the information doctors receive, the symptoms that they observe and the outcomes of the treatment they prescribe are affected by the ways they act and interact with patients (Aspgren, 1999). Equally, there is a need for effective communication skills with members of a healthcare team and the wider community (Bok, 1989; Greenwood, Lewis and Burgess, 1998). Despite this awareness, *practical* courses in communication are but a tiny part of the experience of undergraduate medical students (Hargie *et al*, 1998). It is probable that this finding holds true for intending dentists and veterinary surgeons. The reasons for this lack of emphasis upon communication are the heavily science-based curriculum, the view that 'communication isn't science', the myth that communication skills cannot be taught or, at least, are better picked up as one works with patients (Maguire, 1990), and the perceived marginality of communication to the 'true' purposes of clinical education.

These views are entrenched in the culture although there are signs of change (see Chapter 3 by Jeff Wilson). The change could be accelerated by incorporating early in MDV courses, the experience of working with patients/clients and reflecting on these experiences. Collaborative learning provides opportunities for role modelling of communication and teamwork skills. If these skills are made explicit to the learners then they are likely to be enhanced. More specifically, collegiality and collaborative learning in seminars based on video recording of doctor patient/client consultations are more likely to build self-esteem, confidence and communicative competence than methods of teaching through humiliation (Pendleton *et al*, 1984). Attitudes and techniques of teamwork, mutual supportiveness and mastery of communication and the capacity to work well together are better modelled in a collegial atmosphere than in an authoritarian regime.

The way forward

We are apprehensive about advocating courses of action for the complex issues discussed in this chapter. It is easy to say 'change the culture'. It is difficult to do it – and cultural revolutions often have unexpected consequences. Those who are anxious for practical hints on learning organizations may find useful the text by Day, Peters and Race (1999) but beware of producing superficial solutions to deep problems. Harden (2000) offers two approaches to the future of medical education: possible evolution or revolution. On closer inspection, the evolutionary approach exploits and develops his 'SPICES' curriculum model (Harden *et al*, 1984) and the two revolutionary approaches are both organizational. The first is a suggestion of unitary central control of undergraduate and postgraduate education and the other is the extensive use of virtual delivery. Harden's argument is about methods and neither his evolution nor revolution tips over the dominance of positivistic philosophy. Treating symptoms, and not causes, is not the best way forward although sometimes it is the best that one can do. We do offer the following suggestions for deans, potential deans and other colleagues to consider:

- explore different modes of leadership through seminars and reflective learning tasks;
- look particularly at ways of retaining the best aspects of collegiality in an increasingly bureaucratic world;
- look for ways of persuading international companies and government agencies to support qualitative research on patient care;
- lobby for recognition of qualitative research by the MDV committees of the Research Assessment Exercise;
- encourage more research within MDV Schools on the humanistic aspects of learning to become a doctor and consider the implications of the research for the organization and curriculum of MDV Schools;
- consider incorporating more community-based and patient-centred approaches early in the curriculum in which students are confronted with 'human' as well as 'clinical' problems;
- focus on ways of developing 'detached concern', particularly in clinical courses;
- make greater use of collaborative methods of learning and assessment;
- use more assessment tasks that consider the person (whole animal) in their contexts.

Conclusion

In this chapter we have shown how culture, collegiality and collaborative learning are important considerations for the design and development of learning experiences. Other contributors to this book provide a more detailed exposition of teaching, learning and assessment and cognate matters. We have provided a broad overview in which we have argued that collaborative learning is an essential part of the preparation for MDV students, that collegiality is the foundation for lifelong learning and that the culture of MDV Schools may need to shift towards a more humanistic approach to students. This shift, we argue, will only occur if humanistic as well as scientific research is valued in MDV communities. We have shown that the task is challenging, that there are many tensions to be resolved and many challenges ahead. We end with a quotation from Coles who expresses eloquently the theme of this chapter:

> As curriculum planners and teachers we need to be able to trust our students and trainees more than perhaps we do. They are adults. We must recognise them as such. Our efforts should be directed towards creating the conditions

needed for effective learning, that is by contextualising the educational events we arrange and by supporting our learners in our learning. Nothing more is needed. Nothing less will do. (Coles, 1998: 80)

References

Arluke, A (1980) Roundsmanship: inherent control in a medical teaching ward, *Social Science and Medicine*, **14**, pp 297–302

Aspgren, K (1999) BEME Guide No 2 Teaching and Learning communication skills in medicine – a review with quality grading of articles, *Medical Teacher*, **21**, pp 563–70

Atkinson, P A (1977) The reproduction of medical knowledge, in *Health Care and Health Care knowledge*, eds R Dingwall *et al*, Croom Helm, London

Becher, T and Trowler, P R (2001) *Academic Tribes and Territories: Intellectual enquiries and the cultures of disciplines*, 2nd edn, Open University Press, Buckingham

Becker, H S *et al* (1961) *Boys in White: student culture in medical schools*, University of Chicago Press, Chicago

Biggs, J (1987) *Student Approaches in Learning and Studying*, Australian Council for Educational Research, Hawthorn, Melbourne, Victoria

Biggs, J (1999) *Teaching for quality learning at university: What the student does*, SHRE and Open University Press, Buckingham

Bok, D (1989) Needed: a new way to train doctors, in *New directions for medical education: Problem-based learning and community-oriented medical education*, eds H G Schmidt *et al*, Springer-Verlag, New York

Bowden, J and Marton, F (1998) *The university of learning*, Kogan Page, London

Brown, G and Atkins, M (1988) Understanding the processes of the consultation, *Medical Teacher*, pp 271–78

Brown, G, Bull, J and Pendlebury, M (1997) *Assessing student learning in higher education*, Routledge, London

Bruner, J (1996) *The culture of education*, Harvard University Press, Cambridge, Mass

Burgoyne J (1994) Established and Emergent Learning Company Concepts and Practices, in *The Learning Company: Concepts and Practices*, eds J Boydell, M Pedler and T Boydell, McGraw-Hill, Maidenhead

Coles, C R (1985) Differences between conventional and problem-based curricula in their students' approaches to studying, *Medical Education*, **19**, pp 308–09

Coles, C (1998) The process of learning, in *Medical Education in the Millennium*, eds B Jolly and L Rees, Oxford University Press, Oxford

Cribb, A and Bignold, S (1999) Towards the Reflexive Medical School: the hidden curriculum and medical education research, *Studies in Higher Education*, **24** (2), pp 195–209

Day, A, Peters, J and Race, P (1999) *500 tips for developing a learning organisation*, Kogan Page, London

Dewey, J (1964) *John Dewey on education. Selected writings*, ed and introduction by R D Archambault, University of Chicago Press, Chicago

Dewey, J (1997) *Experience & education*, First Touchstone Edition, New York

Dimitroff, A and Davies, W K (1996) Content Analysis of research in undergraduate medical education, *Academic Medicine*, pp 71, 60–67

Enarson, C and Burg F D (1992) An overview of reform initiatives in medical education 1906 through 1992, *Journal of the American Medical Association*, **268**, pp 1141–43

Entwistle N J and Ramsden P (1983) *Understanding Student Learning*, Croom Helm, London

Entwistle N J and Tait, H (1990) Approaches to Learning: Evaluation of teaching and preferences for contrasting academic environments, *Higher Education*, **19**, pp 169–94

Field, M (1995) *Dental Education at the Crossroads: challenges and change*, National Academy Press, Washington

General Dental Council (GDC) (1997) *The First Five Years*, General Dental Council, London

Genn, J M (2001) AMEE Guide No 23 (Part 1); Curriculum, environment, climate, quality and change in medical education – a unifying perspective, *Medical Teacher*, **23**, pp 337–44

Gentle, P (2001) Course cultures and learning organisations, *Active learning in higher education*, **2** (1), 8–30

General Medical Council (GMC) (1993) *Tomorrow's Doctors*, General Medical Council, London

Greenwood, L F, Lewis, D W and Burgess, R C (1998) How competent do dental graduates feel?, *Journal of Dental Education*, **61**, pp 465–72

Halsey, A H (1992) *The Decline of Donnish Dominion*, Oxford University Press, Oxford

Handy, C (1995) *The age of unreason*, 2nd edn, Arrow Books, London

Harden, R M, Sowden, S and Dunn, W R (1984) Educational strategies in curriculum development: the Spices Model, *Medical Education*, **20**, pp 458–66

Harden, R M (2000) Evolution or revolution and the future of medical education: replacing the oak tree, *Medical Teacher*, **22** (5), pp 435–42

Hargie O *et al* (1998). A survey of communication skills training in UK schools of medicine: present practices and prospective proposals, *Medical Education*, **32**, pp 25–34

ILT (1999) Statement of Professional Values, *Institute of Learning and Teaching* [Online] www.ilt.ac.uk

Jacques, D (2000) *Small Group Teaching*, 3rd edn, Kogan Page, London

Jolly, B (1998) Historical and Theoretical Background, in *Medical Education in the Millennium*, eds B Jolly and L Rees, Oxford University Press, Oxford

Jennett, P (1993) Lifelong self-directed learning, in *Learning in Medicine*, eds C Coles and H A Holm, Scandinavian University Press, Oslo

Jones, S (1996) *Developing a Learning Culture*, McGraw-Hill, Maidenhead

Kogan, M, Moses, I and El-Khawas, E (1994) *Staffing Higher Education*, Kogan Page, London

Kohn, L T, Corrigan, J M and Donaldson, M S (1999) *To err is human*, National Academy Press, Washington DC

Le Fanu, J (1999) *The Rise and Fall of Modern Medicine*, Little Brown and Company, London

Maguire, P (1990) Can communication skills be taught?, *British Journal of Hospital Medicine*, **11**, pp 175–82

Maheux, B *et al* (2000) Medical Faculty as humanistic physicians and teachers: the perceptions at innovative and traditional medical schools, *Medical Education*, **34**, pp 630–34

Manogue, M, Brown, G and Foster H (2001) Clinical assessment of dental students: values and practices of teachers in restorative dentistry, *Medical Education*, **35**, pp 364–70

Newble, D and Clarke, R M (1986) The approaches to learning in traditional and in an innovative medical school, *Medical Education*, **20**, pp 267–73

O'Malley, C D (1970) *The History of Medical Education*, University of California Press, Los Angeles

O'Neill, E H (1992) Education as Part of the Health Care Solution: Strategies from the Pew Health Professions, *Journal of the American Medical Association*, **268** (9), pp 1146–48

Osler, W (1914) *Aequanimitas and Other Addresses to Medical Students, Nurses, and Practitioners of Medicine*, 2nd edn, 3rd impression, P Blakiston & Sons, Philadelphia

Pedler, M (ed) (1991) *Action Learning in Practice*, 2nd edn, Gower, Aldershot

Pedler, M, Burgoyne, J and Boydell, T (1997) *The Learning Company: a strategy for sustainable development*, 2nd edn, McGraw-Hill, Maidenhead

Pendleton, M *et al* (1984) *The Consultation: an approach to learning*, Oxford University Press, Oxford

QAA (2001) *Handbook for Academic Review*, Quality Assurance Agency, Gloucester

Ramsden, P (1992) *Learning to teach in higher education*, Routledge, London

Ramsden, P (1998) *Learning to lead in higher education*, Routledge, London

Ricoeur, P (1981) *Hermeneutics and the Human Sciences*, Cambridge University Press, Cambridge

RCVS (1991) *Report of the Working Party on Veterinary Undergraduate Education* (Chair: J Lucke), Royal College ofVeterinary Surgeons, London

Schmidt H G and Molen, H T (2001) Self-reported competency ratings of graduates of a problem-based medical curriculum, *Academic Medicine*, **76**, pp 466–68

Senge, P M (1992) *The fifth discipline*, Century Business, London

Sinclair, S (1998) *Making doctors: an institutional apprenticeship*, Berg Press, Oxford

Stenhouse, L (1975) An Introduction to Curriculum Research and Development, Heinemann Educational Books, London

Tomasello, M, Kruger, A and Ratner, H (1993) Cultural learning, *Behavioral and Brain Sciences*, **16**, pp 495–511

Trigwell, K, Prosser, M and Waterhouse, F (1999) Relations between teachers' approaches to teaching and students' approaches to learning, *Higher Education*, **37**, pp 57–70

Vincent, D *et al* (2001) Adverse events in British hospitals, *British Medical Journal*, **322**, 517–19

Wilson, V and Pirrie, A (1999) Developing Professional Competence: lessons from the emergency room, *Studies in Higher Education*, **24**, pp 211–24

3

Communication skills: on being patient-centred

Jeff Wilson

Introduction

Why should we all have an interest in learning effective communication skills? Most of us have been communicating since birth and have managed to communicate effectively throughout our lives – or so we think. Communication is a series of learnt skills rather than just natural ability. Some are naturally better at communicating than others. We may all have learnt the ability to interact with people at basic levels, but these skills can be enhanced by both our experience and by education. There is a certain amount of scepticism, almost resentment, when intelligent young adults are obliged to learn communication skills. However, there is overwhelming evidence to suggest that those in the healthcare professions are not as effective at communicating as they would like to think. Research has shown that medical students are poor at discovering patients' main problems and that doctors do not learn to communicate empathically without specific training (Kurtz, Silverman and Draper, 1998). Anecdotal stories of poor interactions with healthcare professionals are common. Doctors who are too busy writing up notes to take much notice of their patients as they enter the surgery. Dentists who proceed straight to the clinical examination and keep their fingers in patients' mouths whilst asking questions. Vets who don't seem interested in what the owners have to say whilst tending to their sick animal.

A great deal of research has been carried out into the need for teaching and learning communication skills. Effective communication skills have been found to make significant differences to a wide range of desirable patient outcomes. Perhaps of more importance is that poor communication is a major factor when patients, relatives or carers express dissatisfaction with care. When the patient is an animal the same is true for its owner, as has been demonstrated by the Veterinary Defence Society in the United Kingdom and the American Veterinary Medical Association (1992). Poor communication can also lead to an increased risk of accidents for the patient and ultimately to litigation. Levinson (1994) found that primary care physicians who used more facilitative statements were less likely to suffer malpractice claims.

Medical education

Research has shown that few doctors currently provide sufficient information for patients to comply with their recommendations (Maguire, Fairbairn and Fletcher, 1986a), or adequately prepare patients for medical interventions (Horne, De and King, 1987). Doctors frequently lack the interactional skills to provide preventive health advice, with many failing to take the first step of detecting the existence of problems among their patients. However, after taking part in communications skills training medical students became more adept at detecting and responding appropriately to patients' verbal and non-verbal cues, and were able to elicit more relevant information from patients (Evans *et al*, 1991).

Historical background

In 1980, the General Medical Council recognized that, on graduation, a medical student should be competent to communicate effectively and sensitively with patients and their relatives. However, a survey of British Medical Schools by Wakeford (1983) found that approximately one-third offered no formal training in communication skills. In 1988, a further study by the General Medical Council found that five schools still did not teach communication skills as a specific entity. In 1992, Fredrikson and Bell published the results of their appraisal of communication skills training in British Medical Schools. They found that, although all survey respondents provided some form of communications skills training, relatively few were committed to formal instruction, assessment and evaluation of the subject within the medical curriculum.

Finally, in *Tomorrow's Doctors* (GMC, 1993) the General Medical Council declared that 'doctors must be good listeners if they are to understand the problems of their patients and they must be able to provide advice and explanations that are comprehensible to patients and their relatives'. It decreed that all Medical Schools must teach communication skills as an integral part of the undergraduate curriculum.

Dental education

Unlike medical undergraduates, dental students actually perform treatment on patients during their training. The General Dental Council (GDC) has recognized that communication skills should be taught as part of the undergraduate curriculum, but only recently. In *The First Five Years* (GDC, 1997), under Skill Objectives it stated: 'the dentist will be able to communicate effectively with patients, their families and associates, and with other health professionals involved with their care'. Under Communication Skills it stated: 'instruction in communication skills is an important aspect of the education of the dental student. As with teaching in psychology and sociology, it can best be undertaken on a collaborative basis by individuals dedicated to the subject and by clinical dental teachers. Initially it may be taught in role-playing situations and with simulated patients. Eventually, however, it will be the basis of students' care of their own patients'.

In the majority of Dental Schools students are taught the theoretical aspects of communication skills, usually as part of their behavioural sciences training in Dental Public Health. They are subsequently expected to learn how to implement these skills in their clinical experience with real patients. Relatively few schools use role play, simulated patients or video feedback at present. However, a survey into the clinical assessment of undergraduate dental students revealed that dental clinical teachers attached great importance to the teaching of communication skills (Manogue, Brown and Foster, 2001).

Veterinary education

Schools of Veterinary Medicine in the United Kingdom have only recently begun to introduce communication skills training into their curricula, but the importance of communication skills for vets has been known for some time (Hendrix, Thompson and Mann, 2001). Not all schools teach this as an integral part of their curriculum, as yet (Eddy, 2001). For example, at Liverpool, a communications skills seminar for fourth-year undergraduates was arranged by the Society of Practising Veterinary Surgeons in 2000. A detailed evaluation of this pilot scheme showed that it proved popular with the students. The Royal College of Veterinary Surgeons have supported this initiative, so it is likely that veterinary communications skills teaching will soon become an integral part of training in all UK Veterinary Schools.

Veterinary communication problems are somewhat different to those of other healthcare disciplines. With animals as their patients, vets must reach a correct diagnosis by first obtaining a history of the problem from the owner before carrying out a physical examination of the patient (Thacher, 1989). For sick animals the vet must not only prescribe and carry out the correct treatment but also must ensure that owners comply with their follow-up instructions.

Breaking bad news

This is a problem for all healthcare professionals. A particular problem for vets is that of euthanasia. To advise someone that their cherished pet is suffering to the point that recovery is unlikely and that the animal should be 'put down' can be a very demanding not to say distressing task for both parties (Turner, 1985). To advise farmers that one or more of their animals should be destroyed has implications of severe financial losses (in addition to the veterinary bill).

Breaking bad news is also a problem for doctors and dentists. It is probably the topic with which most students of communications skills ask for help. The World Health Organisation (1993) recognized that training in breaking bad news helps professionals to deal more effectively with the sensitive aspects of interactions that may be common in practice (Newton and Fiske, 1999) but not usually included in undergraduate training. For example, as we age, our ability to care for ourselves may deteriorate through no fault of our own, eg by debilitating disease such as arthritis, and our health and self-esteem may be adversely affected. The psychological effect that tooth loss can have for certain patients can be deeply distressing and has been likened to bereavement for some people (Fiske, *et al*, 2001).

Communication skills

Whereas generic communication skills can be learnt and developed by all, specific skills are relevant for the individual professions, as in the example of breaking bad news above. Having established that there is a need for learning and teaching communication skills, we should now consider those skills thought necessary for healthcare professionals to acquire. Maguire, Fairbairn and Fletcher (1986b) found that patients who had been interviewed by medical students preferred interviewers who:

- introduced themselves;
- were easy to talk to;
- were warm and sympathetic;
- appeared self-confident;
- listened to them and responded to their verbal cues;
- asked questions which were precise and easily understood;
- did not repeat themselves.

Basic communication skills that can be learnt and developed by all include:

- non-verbal;
- use of questions;
- listening skills;
- use of summaries.

Specific communication skills for MDV professionals include:

- the biomedical and personal agendas;
- the need to involve the patient;
- consultation skills;
- interprofessional skills (including referral).

Non-verbal communication skills, often (inadequately) referred to as 'body language', can have profound effects upon interactions between individuals and between groups. They include

- eye contact;
- posture;
- proximity;
- touch;
- gestures;
- facial expression.

In a study of medical outpatients, a positive relationship was found between patient satisfaction and physician non-verbal communication in the form of physicians' nods and gestures, and closer distance between doctor and patient in the information gathering phase of the consultation. Clinicians who face their patients directly, use more eye contact and maintain an open posture are regarded as more empathic, interested and warm (Weinberger, Greene and Mamlin, 1981).

Use of questions – open and closed

Open questions are general and allow the subject to talk freely – to tell their story. For example, 'What is the problem?' or 'How can I help you?'. Most patients have more than one concern to discuss and the order in which patients present problems is not necessarily related to their clinical symptoms. Beckman and Frankel (1984) showed that patients who are allowed to complete their opening statement without interruption take less than 60 seconds and that the longer doctors wait before interrupting their patients the more problems are elicited. They also showed that even minimal interruptions to opening statements could prevent other important concerns from being discussed.

The advantages of open questioning methods are that they encourage the historian to tell their story in a more complete fashion. They prevent the 'stab in the dark' approach of closed questioning. They allow the questioner time, space to listen, think, and not focus so much on the next question. They contribute to more effective diagnostic reasoning. They help in the exploration of both biomedical and personal agendas and they set a pattern of patient participation rather than clinician domination.

Closed questions are very specific and demand an answer to a particular question – often a single word response. They should be brought in later, as the dialogue develops, where they help in the detection of specific facts that aid diagnosis. For example, 'Does the problem always happen at night?' Closed questions allow the questioner to assume control of the interview. They also tend to pursue a specific line of enquiry. However, they must be used carefully, and can be misleading if they are used too early, with important facts being missed.

Listening skills – the art of active listening

Patients, carers or owners ('clients') don't always say what they mean and often have difficulty in articulating their thoughts. It is important to listen very carefully to what is said, then try to understand what is actually meant or felt. Open questioning styles lead to improved detection of disorders and lead to greater disclosure of significant concerns by clients. It is important to confirm that the listener has understood by either making a supporting statement or reiterating what the patient has said. This technique also allows the client to correct the listener if they have misinterpreted the client's meaning or feelings. It is also important to speak to clients in language they will understand, but without patronizing them (Hadlow and Pitts, 1991).

Use of summaries

Throughout a consultation it is important for the practitioner to show that they have understood what the patient has said. It is also important to have empathized with the client. The art of summarizing is a powerful tool in demonstrating understanding, respect and empathy.

Short summaries should be used at frequent intervals throughout the consultation. They can be very effective when the storyteller comes to a halt and has difficulty finding words to convey their thoughts and feelings. They are thus useful in helping the people to tell their story and in helping the listener convey understanding of what is being thought or experienced. They also give time for clarification of thoughts for both parties. Perhaps more importantly, they leave control of what is said next up to the client. They can also be used to encourage exploration of different lines of thought or even help to examine a problem in a different way. Short summaries have different forms:

- simple repetition of what has just been said;
- rephrasing what has been said;
- extending or interpreting the meaning of what has been said.

Used skilfully, short summaries can become reflective listening statements that form the basis of counselling skills. However, it then becomes important to be careful not to misinterpret what has been said and not to 'put words into the client's mouth'.

Long summaries can be used at key points throughout the consultation. The listener should summarize what has been said in two or three sentences, again giving the storyteller the opportunity to correct misunderstandings. The storyteller should feel that the listener has understood. Both parties can share ideas at this point or fill in the gaps. Here the listener can use more closed questions to clarify important clinical points. Long summaries are often used just before proceeding to the clinical examination. Then, afterwards, they can be used to bring the consultation to a close.

The biomedical and personal agendas

Healthcare professionals generally are very skilled in the biomedical agenda. Students tend to concentrate on this alone. Students feel that it is imperative to establish a correct diagnosis. While this is especially important in the management of the patient's disease, it is only part of the overall story – which can be an important factor in the patient's illness. Students often feel uncomfortable at prying into the more intimate, social side of patients' lives, especially where irrecoverable diseases are involved. For qualified clinicians, failure to obtain a relevant social history can sometimes be due to lack of available time, as well as poor communication skills.

For example, general medical practitioners will complain that under the NHS scheme they have on average only five minutes in which to undertake a consultation. They argue that it is impossible for them to utilize the full range of communication skills in this limited time. Although this argument may be valid and understandable, the inevitable result may be an adverse outcome for some of their patients.

Disease can be defined as the pathological biological process. Illness is the patient's individual experience of this process. The way a patient feels and thinks about their illness and the effects that illness has upon them (and others) can have a profound effect on the prognosis for their management. Practitioners tend to be less adept at establishing the personal agenda. It is important to realize that in order to help patients both the biomedical and personal agendas must be taken into consideration.

The biomedical agenda is the information needed to diagnose and manage a disease that includes signs, symptoms and special investigations. The personal agenda is the client's experience of their illness – their ideas, concerns, expectations, feelings, thoughts and effects. The healthcare professional must understand both the disease and illness experience. This should facilitate finding common ground with the client and lead to shared decision-making. The outcome should be an agreed diagnosis and management plan for the illness rather than the disease alone. The client should also be fully informed so that they will know what is likely to happen next and why. It is therefore important to understand the client's perspective and empathize with them.

The need to involve patients/carers/owners (clients)

Generally, clinicians give sparse information to their clients. Doctors tend to overuse jargon that patients don't understand (Hadlow and Pitts, 1991). Patients do not always comply with treatment plans made by their doctors, with up to 50 per cent not taking prescribed medication correctly (Meichenbaum and Turk, 1987). It is important to realize that negotiation with clients and client participation in decision-making lead to increased adherence to treatment regimens and increased client satisfaction (Eisenthal, Koopman and Stoeckle, 1990).

Consultation skills

The following scheme is modified from the Calgary-Cambridge Guide to *Teaching and Learning Communication Skills in Medicine* (Kurtz, Silverman and Draper, 1998):

- Starting the consultation:
  - establish a rapport;
- Gathering information:
  - explore problems;
  - understand the client's perspective;
- Building the rapport:
  - develop rapport;
  - involve the client;
- Explanation and planning:
  - provide the correct amount and type of information;
  - aid accurate recall and understanding;
  - achieve a shared understanding incorporating the client's perspective;
  - plan future management;
  - share decision-making;
- Closing the consultation:
  - encourage client to discuss any additional points;
  - summaries.

Interprofessional skills – a patient-centred approach

Healthcare is teamwork. Gone are the days of the individual practitioner working alone. Primary, secondary and tertiary care demand effective interprofessional communication. To be able to achieve successful outcomes for clients it is necessary for all members of the healthcare team to be fully informed. That the most important member of the team is the patient is a fact that has often been overlooked! Learner-centred communication skills training can result in allied disciplines working more effectively together.

A clinical referral letter needs to be concise, accurate and justifiable. The biomedical agenda should be reported but the letter may also need to convey that the personal agenda is impacting on the patient's illness whilst, at the same time, maintaining discretion. 'Reading between the lines' cannot always be relied upon to convey the desired meaning (Hodge *et al*, 1992). Any perceived doubts should therefore always be reinforced with unambiguous follow-up, such as a telephone call. There is some evidence to suggest that the overall standard of referral letters is poor (Emmanuel and Walter, 1989; Jenkins, 1993).

Learning and teaching communication skills

When should communication skills be learnt?

There is evidence to suggest that undergraduate medical students become less receptive to communication skills teaching as they progress through their course (Craig, 1992). This is probably because their interest in the biomedical agenda becomes overwhelming (Sanson-Fisher and Poole, 1980). It has therefore been recommended that communication skills should be taught throughout the undergraduate course and that this should continue post-qualification (Bowman *et al*, 1992).

How should communication skills be taught?

A broad spectrum of methods is available for developing communication skills, ranging from didactic teaching through to experiential learning. Teaching methods that have been used successfully to bring about changes in learners' communication skills are handouts, lectures, workshops, role play, simulated patients, real patients and the use of video and audio recordings for feedback.

Knowledge of communication skills does not translate directly to improved performance. Experiential learning is required to allow the acquisition of new skills, but perhaps more importantly to change the learners' behaviour (Kurtz, Silverman and Draper, 1998). For all aspects of learning the student must not only want to learn but must also feel a need to learn for self-improvement. It is therefore of paramount importance to enable students to realize that they can learn to communicate more effectively, thereby awakening an interest in the subject and stimulating their willingness to learn.

Communication skills learning and teaching requires one-to-one or small group learning in which the individual learner can have frequent opportunity for practice, participation and individual coaching. (Kurtz, Silverman and Draper, 1998). An introduction to basic communication skills can be didactic, for example in the form of lectures, but this should quickly move on to experiential learning in which small group working plays an important part. Simple, non-clinical exercises can be attempted by large groups subdivided into smaller working groups. This can then be followed by feedback firstly in small groups and then the large group as a whole. The role of facilitator is crucial when dealing with large groups in the control and direction of the ordered session.

Progression can then be made to small groups working with video feedback using simulated patients. The advantages of video feedback are: self-assessment, learner involvement, objectivity, accuracy, specificity of feedback, description with analysis of behaviour, and a permanent record that can be revisited. At first learners may find the thought of video feedback of their performance in front of their peers uncomfortable, even threatening. Most are initially reluctant. However, the use of video recordings to guide feedback offers many advantages over feedback from simple observations by a third party. Again, the role of facilitator is crucial in setting the ground rules for the small group session. Learners should feel comfortable. The advantages of using video feedback must be explained. Feedback should emphasize the positive whilst dealing sensitively with negative comments, both from the learner and their peers. It is interesting to note that individuals tend to be hypercritical of their own performance whilst their peers tend to be very supportive and only mildly critical of even the most disastrous performances!

Simulated patients

Simulated patients enable learners to practice their communication skills in a relatively safe and non-threatening environment. The use of simulated patients has been shown to be effective, reliable and valid for both learning and assessment of communication skills (Vu and Barrows, 1994). Well-trained simulated patients can be so effective that students and practising doctors cannot distinguish between them and real patients (Sanson-Fisher and Poole, 1980).

Originally, simulated patients for communication skills teaching were recruited from real patients who had experienced the illnesses they presented. Now they tend to be professional (or semi-professional) actors specially trained for the purpose. This does add to the expense of organizing a course but their advantages more than outweigh their drawbacks. Medical students realize that they are in role play situations and are not as worried about incorrect diagnoses or the potential for causing harm to a real patient. Dental and veterinary students gain by experiential learning – a definite advantage that would be ethically unacceptable for medical students.

Feedback

Didactic teaching alone is not successful when attempting to teach communication skills. Experiential learning is the key to success. However, it does have certain problems associated with it. Learners initially find it more challenging and less comfortable than didactic teaching. Criticism, whether by self or from one's peers, is rarely easy to accept and the existence of a video recording of the actual performance exposes the learners to revisiting their mistakes as well as their successes.

Experiential learning is less structured in that there is no script. The simulated patients follow guidelines as to their presenting condition but can and should be encouraged to improvise. As a result, sometimes even the best of students can be lost for words. Also, in small group learning each member of the group will have a different style of learning as well as a different level of knowledge and therefore different needs. The facilitator has a crucial role to play in ensuring that each session is structured in such a way that, whilst adhering to the curriculum, the environment is as safe and non-threatening as possible. For this reason ground rules for feedback have been developed (Pendleton *et al*, 1984):

- briefly clarify matters of fact;
- self-assessment first – the learner being observed gives a critical appraisal of their own performance;
- the rest of the group are then given the opportunity to comment on what was done well and how;
- the learner then says what could be improved or done differently and how;
- the facilitator and the rest of the group then make suggestions as to how the interview could have been done differently.

Students tend to be hypercritical of their own performance and are more sensitive to criticism from their peers than from teachers. It is important to emphasize positive aspects initially and then deal with negative self-criticism by recommendations for improvement rather than agreeing with the negative aspects or appearing judgemental. It is important that the whole group is involved in feedback. The group can work to generate solutions to problems that not only will help the learner but will also help themselves when they encounter similar situations.

Who should teach and train?

The World Summit on Medical Education (1993) recommended that teaching staff competent in communication skills teaching (not necessarily clinicians) should become core trainers of a broad range of teachers drawn from a wide variety of clinical specialities. These teachers would then support the training of undergraduate students in communication skills and ensure that the skills learnt are reinforced throughout the curriculum.

Assessment of communication skills

Why assess?

Evaluation motivates students to learn, legitimizes the importance of the subject to students and encourages acceptance of the subject by academic staff (Kurtz, Silverman and Draper, 1998). Both formative and summative methods of assessment should be used in the assessment of communication skills.

Formative assessment should facilitate learning in a non-judgemental, non-threatening environment. It is ongoing and takes place throughout training. Both teachers and learners should be involved. For communication skills, an important aim of formative assessment is to encourage learners to engage in honest and open self-assessment to the point of admitting and discussing their own difficulties.

Summative assessment traditionally is in the form of examinations at set times throughout the course. Undergraduates tend to become focussed on summative assessments, as progression through the course is usually conditional on passing these assessments. The case can therefore be made for including summative assessments as an integral part of the communication skills course for example, by linking it with the clinical skills examinations. This has two advantages: it links the practical importance of communication skills with the history and examination of real patients and it assigns the importance necessary for learners to want to improve their communication skills (Westberg and Jason, 1993).

Who should assess?

As communication skills learning is essentially experiential, formative assessment should be dominant. Both self-assessment and peer assessment are of considerable importance in formative assessments. The ability to self-assess is essential for lifelong learning in clinical practice (Hays, 1990). It is therefore important for the learner to be involved in their own assessments (Farnill, Hays and Todisco, 1997). Also feedback from real and/or simulated patients can be valuable (Spencer *et al*, 2000).

How should students be assessed?

The objective structured clinical examination (OSCE) using simulated patients with video feedback is becoming widely used in the summative assessment of competence in communication skills. Vu and Barrows (1994) have demonstrated the validity, reliability and feasibility of using this method of assessment.

Feedback

Feedback should be given despite the assessment being summative. To simply tell learners that they have either passed or failed and can or cannot progress to the next summative hurdle is of little value for their experiential learning. Feedback on knowledge, competence, performance and outcome should be given as soon after the assessment as is practicably possible. Although examiners may be anonymous, their marking scheme should be according to set criteria and available to learners. Explanatory comments should support both negative and positive marking.

Conclusion

Although all healthcare disciplines now realize the importance of teaching communication skills, the vast majority of research into this subject has been in medical education. It is encouraging to note that there has been a lot of development for postgraduate communication skills teaching over the past few years, but undergraduate teaching seems varied in content, timing, duration and assessment amongst the different schools, with inadequate resources and lack of trained staff being cited as the main problems (Hargie *et al*, 1998).

The same appears to be happening with veterinary education, ie, the emphasis on improving communication skills being seen as important for clinicians post-qualification rather than undergraduate students. As mentioned earlier, not all Veterinary Schools teach communication skills as part of their undergraduate curriculum.

Dentistry is somewhat different to medicine in that communication skills teaching, whilst recognized as important, is not given the same emphasis in the undergraduate curriculum. Perhaps this is because dental students are trained by actively treating patients and are expected to acquire effective communication skills soon in the course, whilst medical and veterinary students don't assume responsibility for their own patients until after qualification.

Whatever the discipline it is obvious that learning communication skills definitely improves the effectiveness of clinicians and improves the outcomes for patients:

- Communication is a learned set of skills.
- Communication skills need to be taught professionally.
- Clinical communication skills are professional skills with specific subject areas that need to be developed by experiential learning.
- Communication skills teaching and learning:
  - is different;
  - is difficult;
  - should be evidence-based;
  - should be experiential;
  - should be a continuous lifelong process.

I am grateful to Dr Paul Kinnersley, Dr Steve Rollnick and to Mrs Josie Manley of the Department of General Practice, University of Wales College of Medicine, for inviting me to participate in their communication skills course. For this course they have drawn heavily on the Calgary-Cambridge *Guide to Teaching Communication Skills in Medicine*, as adapted by Kurtz, Silverman and Draper (1998) in their book *Teaching and Learning Communication Skills in Medicine*. I would recommend this text to anyone with an interest in teaching and learning communication skills. I would also like to thank Professor Sandy Love (Glasgow) and Dr Alan Radford (Liverpool) who have informed me of the current status of communication skills teaching in veterinary medicine in the United Kingdom.

References

American Veterinary Medical Association (1992) Communicate to avoid malpractice claims, *Journal of the American Veterinary Medical Association*, **201** (3), p 383

Beckman, H B and Frankel, R M (1984) The effect of physician behaviour on the collection of data, *Annals of Internal Medicine*, **101**, pp 692–96

Bowman, F M *et al* (1992) Improving the skills of established general practitioners: the long-term benefits of group teaching, *Medical Education*, **26**, pp 63–68

Craig, J L (1992) Retention of interviewing skills learned by first year medical students: a longitudinal study, *Medical Education*, **26**, pp 276–81

Eddy, R G (2001) Communication skills training, *Veterinary Record*, **148** (10), p 320

Eisenthal, S, Koopman, C and Stoeckle, J D (1990) The nature of patients' requests for physicians' help, *Academic Medicine*, **65**, pp 401–05

Emmanuel, J and Walter, N (1989) Referrals from general practice to hospital outpatient departments: a strategy for improvement, *British Medical Journal*, **299**, pp 722–24

Evans, B J *et al* (1991) Effects of communication skills training on students' diagnostic efficiency, *Medical Education*, **25**, pp 517–26

Farnill, D, Hays, S C and Todisco, J (1997) Interviewing skills: self-evaluation by medical students, *Medical Education*, **31**, pp 122–27

Fiske, J *et al* (2001) The emotional effects of tooth loss in partially dentate people attending prosthodontic clinics in dental schools in England, Scotland and Hong Kong: a preliminary investigation, *International Dental Journal*, **51**, pp 457–62

Frederikson, L and Bell, P (1992) An appraisal of the current status of communication skills training in British medical schools, *Social Science & Medicine*, **34** (5), pp 515–22

General Dental Council (GDC) (1997) *The First Five Years: The Undergraduate Dental Curriculum*, General Dental Council, London

General Medical Council (GMC) (1980) *Recommendations as to Basic Medical Education*, General Medical Council, London

GMC (1988) *Report of a Survey of Medical Education Practices in United Kingdom Medical Schools*, General Medical Council, London

GMC (1993) *Tomorrow's Doctors*, General Medical Council, London

Hadlow, J and Pitts, M (1991) The understanding of common terms by doctors, nurses and patients, *Social Science & Medicine*, **32**, pp 193–96

Hargie, O *et al* (1998), A survey of communication skills training in UK schools of medicine: present practices and prospective proposals, *Medical Education*, **32** (1), pp 25–34

Hays, R B (1990), Assessment of general practice consultations: content validity of a rating scale, *Medical Education*, **24**, pp 110–16

Hendrix, C M, Thompson, I K and Mann, C J (2001), A survey of reading writing and oral communication skills in North American Veterinary Medical Colleges, *Journal of Veterinary Medical Education*, **28** (1), pp 34–40

Hodge, J A H *et al* (1992) Medical clinic referral letters. Do they say what they mean? Do they mean what they say?, *Scottish Medical Journal*, **37** (6), pp 179–80

Horne, D, De, L and King, N L (1987) Preparation for surgery, in *Health Care: a behavioural approach*, ed N J King and A Remenyi, pp 167–73, Grune and Stratton, Sydney

Jenkins, R M (1993) Quality of general practitioner referrals to outpatient departments: assessment by specialists and a general practitioner, *British Journal of General Practice*, **43** (368), pp 111–13

Kurtz, S M, Silverman, J and Draper, J (1998) *Teaching and Learning Communication Skills in Medicine*, Radcliffe Medical Press, Abingdon, UK

Levinson, W (1994) Physician-patient communication: a key to malpractice prevention, *Journal of the American Medical Association*, **272** (20), pp 1619–20

Maguire, G P, Fairbairn, S and Fletcher, C (1986a) Consultation skills of young doctors II: Most young doctors are bad at giving information, *British Medical Journal*, **292**, pp 1576–78

Maguire, G P, Fairbairn, S and Fletcher, C (1986b) Consultation skills of young doctors I: Benefits of feedback training in interviews as students persist, *British Medical Journal*, **292**, pp 1573–76

Manogue, M, Brown, G and Foster, H (2001) Clinical assessment of dental students: values and practices of teachers in restorative dentistry, *Medical Education*, **35**, pp 364–70

Meichenbaum, D and Turk, D C (1987) *Facilitating treatment adherence: a practitioner's guidebook*, Plenum Press, New York

Newton, J T and Fiske, J (1999) Breaking bad news: a guide for dental healthcare professionals, *British Dental Journal*, **186**, pp 278–81

Pendleton D *et al* (1984) *The consultation: an approach to learning and teaching*, Oxford University Press, Oxford

Proceedings of the World Summit on Medical Education (1993), *Medical Education*, **28**, Supplement 1, pp 142–49

Sanson-Fisher, R W and Poole, A D (1980) Simulated patients and the assessment of students' interpersonal skills, *Medical Education*, **14**, pp 249–53

Spencer, J *et al* (2000) Patient-oriented learning: a review of the role of the patient in the education of medical students, *Medical Education*, **34** (10), pp 851–57

Thacher, C (1989) Problems with owner communications, *Problems in Veterinary Medicine*, **1** (3), pp 478–90

Turner, T (1985) The unexpected death – how well do we communicate, *Veterinary Record*, **117** (15), p 371

Vu, N V and Barrows, H (1994) Use of standardised patients in clinical assessments: recent developments and measurement findings, *Educational Researcher*, **23**, pp 23–30

Wakeford, R (1983) Communication skills training in United Kingdom medical schools, in *Doctor-Patient Communication*, eds D Pendleton and J Hasler, pp 233–47, Academic Press, London

Weinberger, M, Greene, J Y and Mamlin, J J (1981) The impact of clinical encounter events on patient and physician satisfaction, *Social Science & Medicine*, **15E** (3), pp 239–44

Westberg, J and Jason, H (1993) *Collaborative clinical education: the foundation of effective healthcare*, Springer, New York

World Health Organisation (WHO) (1993) *Doctor-patient interaction and Communication*, World Health Organisation, WHO/MNH/PSF/93.11

4

Curriculum

John Sweet

Introduction

This chapter starts with the hypothetical scenario of two applicants for places at an MDV School. The students apply and enter the school successfully and their progress is followed as the chapter unfolds.

Students' learning and experiences are the most important aspects of a successful curriculum, together with successful communication and adaptation to a caring professional culture. The contrasting traditional and modern problem-based curricula are compared with an all-stakeholders model, which places the community of students, patients, teachers and co-professionals at centre stage. A philosophy of taking every opportunity for learning is advocated. Four contenders are suggested as possible extreme or dominating modes of teaching as lecture-based, virtual-based, problem-based and competency-based. All these approaches offer valuable learning potential, but favouring just one approach to the exclusion of the others does not appear to be supported by the available evidence.

MDV educational environment and curriculum

Applicant scenarios: who is the better candidate?

Jack has always wanted to be a doctor/dentist/vet from the time he first visited his father's group practice in the local town centre. He is an affable well-spoken lad and has been particularly successful in various sports at school. He feels lucky that he has had the opportunity to go to a well-equipped independent school where class sizes have always been very small and where he can also get extra tutoring when needed. Through his father's colleagues he has visited hospital and community clinics over the years. He has become a team leader in the school's voluntary support scheme where students elect to visit and help the elderly. The girl of his life at the moment is Jill.

Jill is from a second generation Caribbean family and attends a large urban comprehensive school. She is one year younger than Jack but they hope to apply to MDV School at the same time. Jill is particularly studious and has done remarkably well at GCSEs and is predicted to do well at A level and the Vocational Training exams she has chosen as well. Apart from enjoying tennis, where she met Jack, she is an outgoing person who makes the most of her part-time job at Burger King, meeting all sorts. She has been uncertain of what she wanted to do until a year or so ago when she undertook various work experiences. She tried out physiotherapy, optometry and even a bank job as well as MDV and having made up her mind has visited two MDV Schools as well as a practice and community clinic.

Despite the large number of sons and daughters who do follow their parents' footsteps into the MDV professions, children are not quite born to the MDV professions! In fact, with the current climate of avoiding discrimination and furthering fairness I use the two scenarios of Jack and Jill at Dental School careers open days to make the point that from the information given both are equally good applicants. I have made reference to MDV for the purpose of this book. Hidden in the text is the likely story that Jack has to resit so that entry requirements may be higher for him. Also, I would include the friendly advice that not all universities are the same and that some would not consider resit applicants or give any credit for vocational training qualifications.

Questions for a potential applicant

- What is your vision? Why would you like to do MDV?
- What A levels or equivalent are you doing and what grades do you think you will get? Have you needed to resit any?
- What have you done or what are your interests that would support your application to become a doctor/dentist/vet?
- What work experience have you done and how have you investigated the MDV professions or career alternatives?
- What reasons have you for choosing a particular school?
- Do you think you will be interviewed for a place here? What do you think the interview will be like?

In addition, I give out a self-questionnaire (above). The questions touch base with fundamental issues of entering professional life successfully. Clearly, there is a tremendous commitment in terms of time and effort so that the student must be highly motivated and obtain the academic entry requirements. In MDV Schools, student learning occurs in multiple specialist environments so that work experience is vital for the student to be able to refine down their preferences to make a choice of profession. The influence of local conditions can also be critical for successful learning. The interview is conducted mainly to assure the school that these considerations have been made, so Jack and Jill will be retained successfully within the course, qualify and continue lifelong learning to the end of their professional lives.

When students are admitted to the MDV School they enter a new learning environment (see Figure 4.1). Genn (2001: 337) emphasizes that those managing the school should appreciate how students perceive this environment. He designates these collective perceptions as the educational climate. In the early years, students are also greatly influenced by the teachers who aim to help them understand how to learn and facilitate learning. The overall context is largely determined for the students by the learning organization through the curriculum.

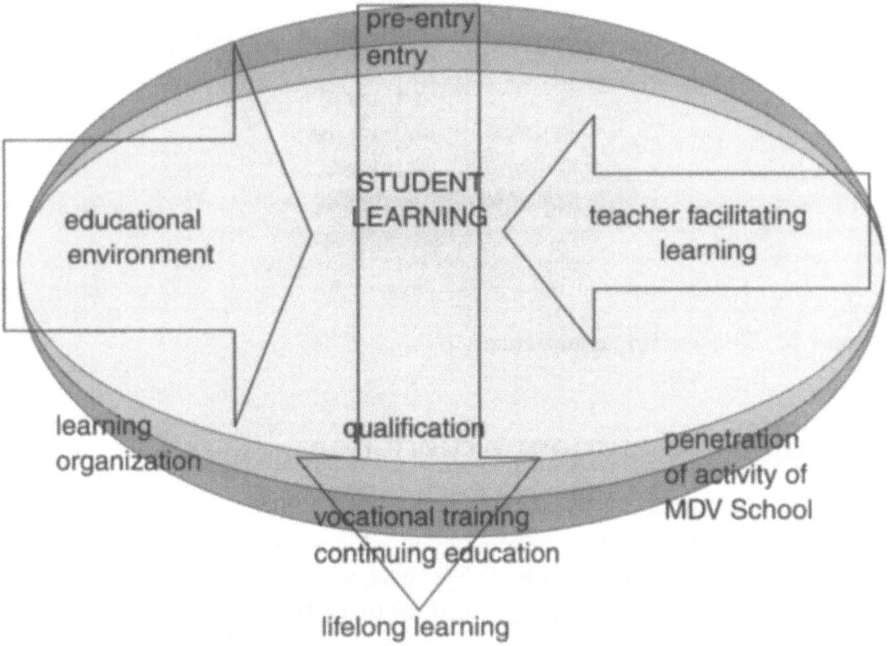

Figure 4.1 MDV Educational context

Looking at the curriculum

Views on what curriculum means have varied from a narrow 'syllabus' or 'just the content' view to one that includes 'all the student experiences inside or outside the school' (Kerr, 1968). This second view was quite a breakthrough in thinking because it replaced the outmoded view that education is largely about the transmission of knowledge from the teacher to student as an empty receptacle. Kerr's position has a student focus. There is a profound interest in Jack and Jill as learners and how their learning is managed as well as the overall learning environment and what is taught and how it is taught. In addition, this approach acknowledges the 'hidden curriculum' – the values and patterns of behaviour that are acquired often incidentally (Harden, 2001). However, some medical curriculum planners have favoured a definition that only includes the planned intended events (Kern, Thomas and Howard, 1998) whilst Socket (1976) emphasizes the importance of the student/teacher relationship and the activities generated by them.

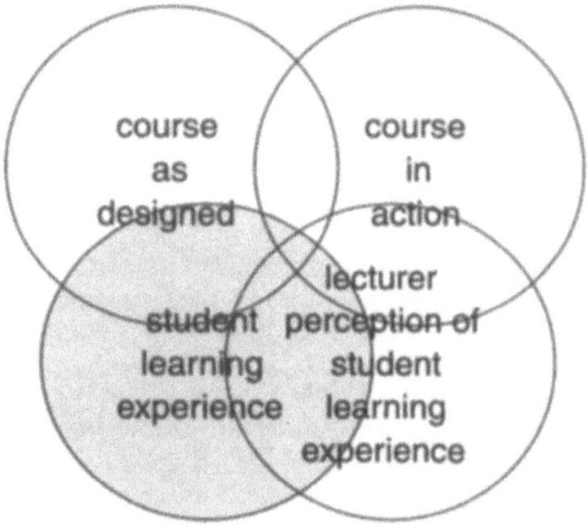

Figure 4.2 The learning experience

Curriculum as student experience

Whatever is planned in the curriculum on paper will differ from what actually takes place. Figure 4.2 shows a circle model developed from Coles (1977), which indicates the potential for curriculum drift, where student experience begins to differ more and more from what is planned for them. It is also useful to note that the teachers' perceptions of the student experience may well be quite different again. It is therefore important to ensure that there is continual student feedback even from distant outposts of clinical placement learning. Genn (2001), however, would include all four circles and more in his definition of curriculum that includes 'all that is happening in a [MDV] School'. This definition places the curriculum within a wider context and some of the various curricular elements are placed in Figure 4.3. The diagram shows the complexity of a modern university, which Habermas (1992) says is a 'bundle institution'. The bundling of functions includes general education and specific training, the research process, assessment, accreditation and setting of standards and also issues in ethics and policy within society, development of culture, self-development and reflective practice.

Community, communication and student learning

Communication is the essential feature that permits these various roles to function together. The MDV university is also a wide-based community of staff and students. The main feature shown in Figure 4.3 is the emphasis on students and student learning. Learning to learn is an important interest because it is acknowledged that much of current professional practice will become outmoded and inappropriate in just a few years. Although what is learnt and how it is learnt is important, no longer is there an obsession with content – for soon much of it may be valueless. Self-development of students to work with change and develop new skills continually for the rest of their lives must be a focus for the planned educational experience.

Student learning and professional mentality – Kolb's learning cycle

A greater understanding of how a clinical student learns and the role of the clinical teacher can be achieved by considering Kolb's (1984) learning cycle at an individual level (see also Chapter 11).

The vertical axis represents concrete experience and abstract conceptualization, which are diametrically opposite methods of 'grasping' or taking hold of an experience. The horizontal axis of reflective observation and active experimentation represents two opposite methods of transforming the 'grasped' experience into a potent and lasting learning experience. In the first instance students must be able to involve themselves fully, openly and without bias in new experiences, ie, concrete experience. They must be able to reflect on their experiences from many perspectives, ie, reflective observation. They must be able to create concepts that integrate observations into logically sound models, ie, abstract conceptualization, and they must be able to use these models to make decisions, solve problems or generally improve complex situations by active experimentation.

Different individuals are likely to favour one or more of these modes. For instance, Jill may be a more outgoing active type, spending more time doing things, whereas Jack might be spending more time reflecting on his experiences. This

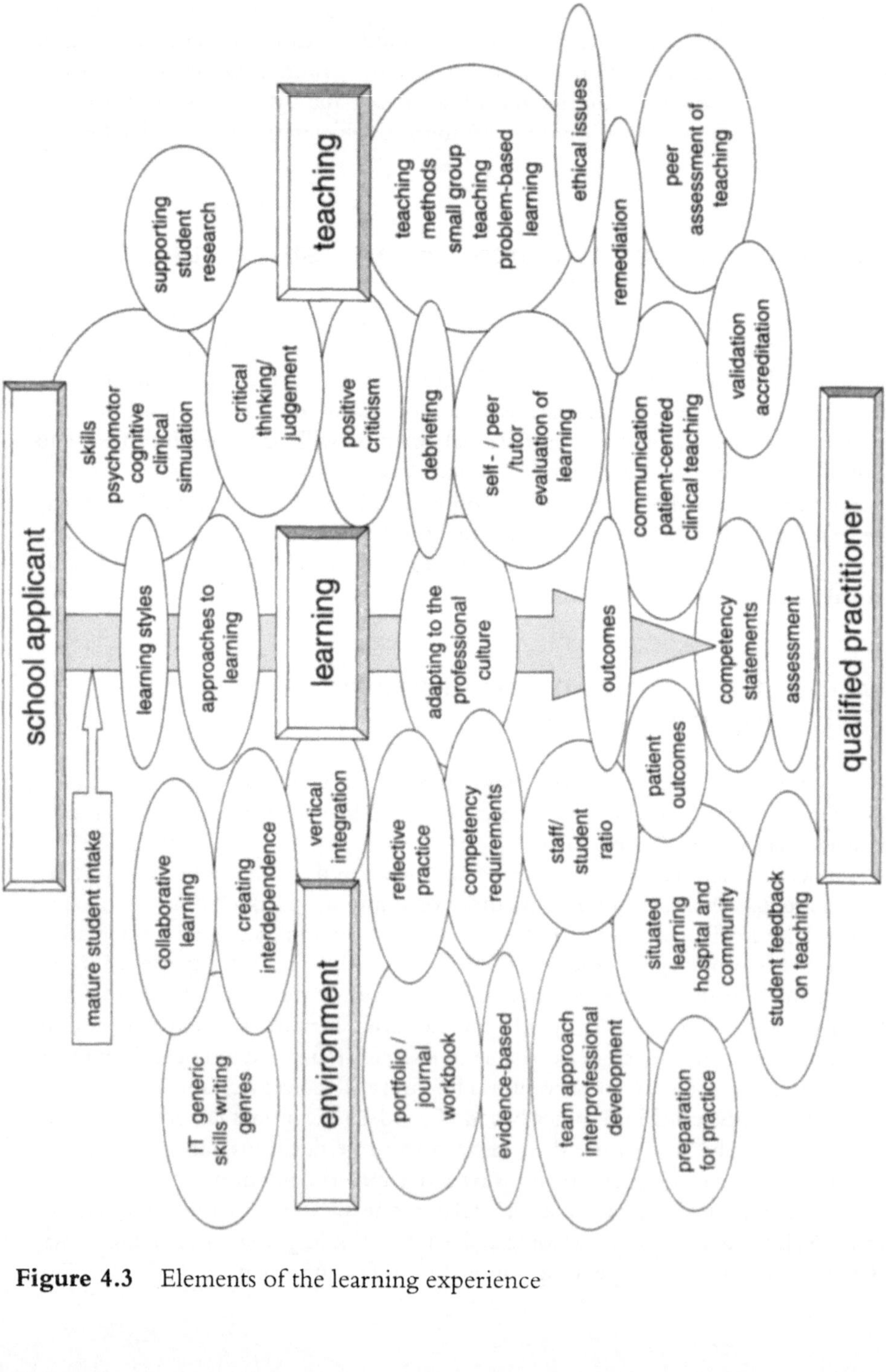

Figure 4.3 Elements of the learning experience

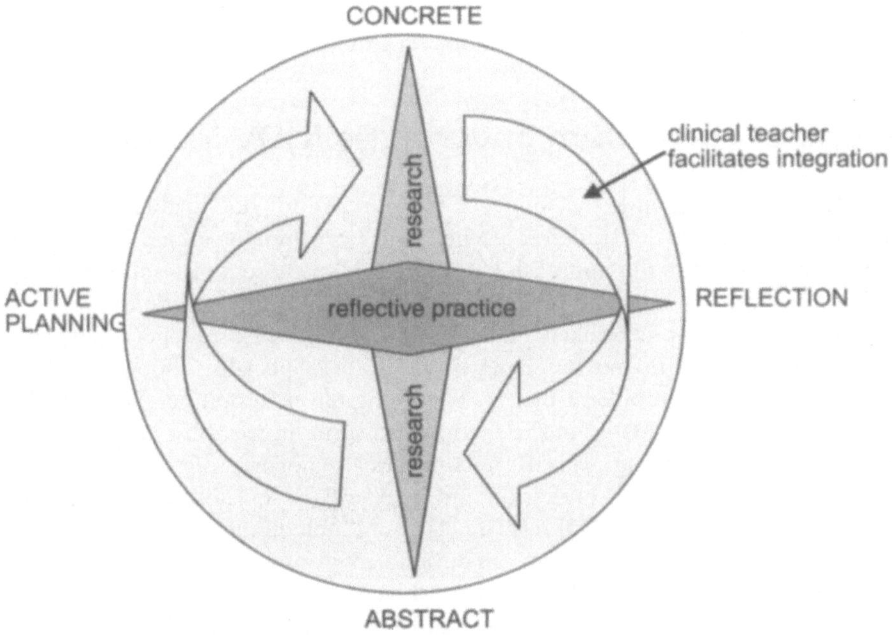

Figure 4.4 Reflective practice, research and clinical teaching after Kolb (1984)

learning theory can also be applied to the professions as a whole, which tend to shape attitudes and orientations towards learning, so much so, that Kolb is concerned about what he terms professional deformation. He proposes that over-learning of a specialized professional mentality may actively hinder adaptation to the changing requirements of an individual's career. If Jill's curriculum and professional mentality are almost exclusively orientated to basic sciences and performing of a range of technological procedures, she may find herself unprepared and inflexible if she advances in her career to become leader of a mixed professional health team. Kolb (1984) was therefore one of the first to attempt to stem the tide of over-specialization and encourage development of more generic skills such as writing and communication.

In MDV education the situation is complex. In 'basic science' subjects the nature of learning inquiry (ie, research) is such that there is a continual grasping toward the concrete and towards the abstract, with fewer demands for reflection or for action planning shown in Figure 4.4. This contrasts greatly with clinical practice. Here the emphasis is upon reflecting on the data available clinically and in the literature, in order to produce a diagnosis and appropriate plan of action. This activity can also be shown in Figure 4.4 as a horizontally placed axis of transformation, towards the reflective pole as integrated inquiry and towards the active pole as treatment solution. In this context the major role of the MDV lecturer is to facilitate well-rounded student learning for academic and clinical life. In Kolb's learning terms, the aim is to produce self-directed persons who are highly developed in each of the learning modes: active, reflective, abstract and concrete. It is then that they may experience tension and conflict that leads to creativity.

Scope of curriculum beyond the MDV institution

Bertolami (2001) extends the range of the curriculum still further to all that shown in Figure 4.1: the students, teachers and environment in and beyond the university. He justifies this approach by stating that many schools cannot keep up to date with the teaching and technical advances that go on outside the schools. Teaching should respond to likely practice demands for when students qualify and, in addition, prepare students for change in the future. Specialists should carry out the tasks and clinical problems that are becoming fewer in number. Some of this training could be conducted in the schools and some in specialist centres where the innovations are taking place. Bertolami sees a major role of the schools is to introduce students to their profession and help student socialization (or reacculturation to use Bruffee's [1993] term). This could include the kind of adjustment that Jack would have to make from the didactic environment of public school to a greater degree of self-directed learning at university. Those adjustments could be just as difficult as the changes in culture and values that Jill may have to make to join the MDV professions.

Other opportunities Bertolami sees for development are possibilities for individual students to complete courses in a time span that matches their skills and learning style, which he calls an asynchronous model. Jack and Jill may start the course together but on past performance Jill would be likely to finish sooner in this model. Some of the specific innovations suggested here may prove difficult to implement but the emphasis on the widest possible interpretation of curriculum appears valuable in developing a workable model for MDV curricula.

Harden, Sowden and Dunn (1984) have set out the SPICES strategy as a progressive approach to curricular development for medical education (see Figure 4.5). They contrast a traditionally taught course with their suggested alternatives. The traditional curriculum is lecture-based and so teacher-centred. The material is taught in disciplines with a standard content and teaching takes place centrally in a large teaching hospital using the resources that are available. They present SPICES as an enlightened alternative. They declared this curriculum to be student-centred and problem-based rather than lecture-based. The content is integrated into themes rather than being taught by separate disciplines with much conducted in community-based placements. One of the features of the curriculum is the development of a standardized compulsory core content that students can supplement with optional elective projects. This changing polarization towards students' learning appeared to be such a fundamental difference, especially with the use of problem-based learning, that curricula were named 'problem-based' to contrast them with traditional forms.

Traditional didactic	Problem-based
teacher-centred lecture-based taught in disciplines hospital-based standardized content taught using available resources	S student-centred P problem-based I integrated into themes C community-based E elective optional plus core content S systematic organization (SPICES after Harden, 1984)

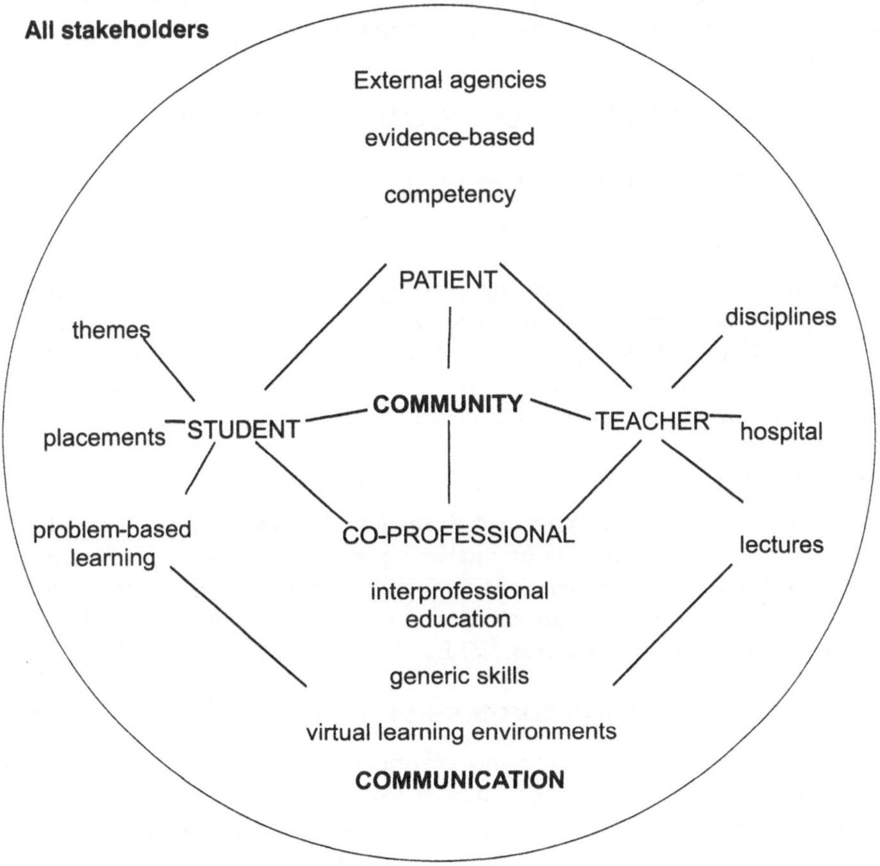

Figure 4.5 Curriculum models

Since 1984, the concept of the curriculum has widened and become far more complex so that this simplistic polarity of student- or teacher-based learning appears less appropriate. A number of new players now have considerable impact on curriculum. Firstly, there are the direct influences of external agencies that represent the interests of patients, and systems, which universities put into place to assure themselves and those agencies that standards of care are reached and maintained. Secondly, there has been a massive expansion of electronic communication and information, with the possibilities of forming virtual learning environments (VLEs). Thirdly, there is recognition that many generic skills, especially those involved with communication, are a necessary part of university education. Finally, there is a recent realization that working in teams with other health professionals is an essential aspect of good clinical practice and should therefore also be an essential aspect of good clinical teaching. A realistic and workable curriculum is one that takes account of all these influences, but does not lose touch with the human side of nurturing the individual student experience.

All-stakeholders curriculum model

Figure 4.5 above also illustrates the all-stakeholders MDV curriculum model:

Community

Community here refers to the collective group of students, teachers, other health professionals and support staff, patients and their carers who interact with the student inside the MDV organization or wherever the student is placed. (This contrasts with the use of the term community-based in the SPICES model that refers to community placements outside the main teaching hospital.)

Communication

Communication with some purpose is essential within the community at all levels and with all members. This can be vital at a personal level between student and patient and student and teacher as well as other members of the healthcare team. Also important for learning are electronic means of communication between students and teacher and student and VLE.

Generic skills and interprofessional education

Critical thinking, active listening and writing skills, given here as examples of generic skills, are required by all health professionals who need to work together as a team when they qualify. It is therefore appropriate that students from different disciplines and professions learn together to work together.

Patient

A focus on the patient in the curriculum can be achieved by stipulating that trainee clinicians will have to develop skills and knowledge to preset standards – they will have to show competency. A further requirement is that clinicians will respect the needs and values of patients and should, where possible, prescribe treatments that are based on sound clinical evidence.

Teacher

The teacher is shown on the right of Figure 4.5, and has been traditionally connected to a discipline, is hospital-based and gives lectures. In the problem-based model, teachers collaborate to set the learning materials for students. In the all-stakeholders model, the teacher is collaborating with other professionals, communicating using information technology and considering how the interests of patients can be safeguarded in the educational process.

Student

The traditional student would attend lectures delivered in discrete disciplines at a main teaching hospital. In the problem-based model, content is arranged seamlessly in themes as they relate to patient case scenarios and learning in placements outside the main hospital is encouraged. In the all-stakeholders model, students will be learning and working in a very wide-ranging environment with other health professionals sharing generic and joint subject interests. They could be following systematically themed problems in a core competency-based course or alternatively follow optional specialist projects. They will be continually using information technology to evidence information, to contact colleagues and teachers. The all-stakeholders curriculum would advocate a flexible approach of taking every opportunity for learning, a willingness to take calculated risks, whether with attempted friendships and collaborations or with the use of new technology. Despite the complexity, individual students still inhabit a space in this model. It is possible to envisage Jack working on a generic healthcare skill issue such as infection control with a student co-professional such as a nurse using problem-based learning. Aware of competency that she must show as a health professional, a further picture of Jill at the computer screen can be conjured, searching for evidence about the best treatment for a patient she has just seen with a rare condition. She may then decide to take a special interest in the treatment modality, for instance, as an elective project. Working within such a community there can be no one overriding dominating component.

Extreme curricula – lecture-, problem-, virtual- and competency-based

There are probably no longer the resources available in most MDV Schools to have the luxury of what Bowden and Marton (1998) call extreme curricula, which try to conduct teaching exclusively using one mode or principle. They identify three possible dogmas as the traditional lecture-based, problem-based and most recently virtual-based learning. To this should be added competency-based. All extreme approaches, if enforced as a chosen method of teaching, may prevent teachers from making professional judgements about how they can enhance appropriate learning for their students as individuals.

Each of these potential mono-curricula will be considered in turn. Each mode or method has distinct advantages associated with it, and these can be brought into the all-stakeholders model.

Lectures

Lectures have been used in traditional courses as a blanket means of 'delivery' of a body of knowledge to the students who are passively receptive. But it does not have to be like that (see Chapter 6). Lectures can be a good introduction to a subject, and do not have to be 'stand alone'; they can be followed by seminars and other group activities that may be more conducive to learning. For this reason, lectures may be most useful to give a taste of a subject; to inform rather than for facilitating general learning of a body of knowledge.

Another place for lectures may be where participants already know the subject quite well. Students may find it difficult to find an up-to-date appraisal of a specialist topic and could make a request for a lecturer to give a presentation on this. Postgraduate students in particular may want to know the specific views of named experts in their field and would be able to identify various aspects of the presentation and be well placed to ask relevant questions for clarification. From a student point of view there is a positive aspect that lectures enable an equitable availability of teachers. Small group teaching always produces insecurity for some students who feel that their group may not have access to as good handouts or tutor as another group.

From a competency-based view, the primary lecturer function is to ensure that all students, with very few exceptions, will reach the required standards in core subjects. With this approach it is unsatisfactory to give students equal attention and let the student-learning settle into the usual bell curve. Instead, every effort is made to draw those failing students up through extra tuition or remediation. Jack may be struggling to understand the content of a lecture, and whilst given the opportunity to ask questions, may not be able to articulate them following a lecture. Back-up, with access to handouts or Web-based postings may or may not help. He may do better to have a small group discussion with Jill!

Virtual learning environments (VLEs)

It has been argued that the enthusiasm for virtual learning environments in higher education generally is almost entirely commercially driven (Delanty, 2001) so that a participating university becomes no more than a producer of educational products. It promotes centralization because the materials are produced and held by the university. Delanty says this creates a polarization of genuine lecturer and student educational interests versus the commercial exploitation of the university. Others see information technology as a means of revolutionary change to improve and augment learning with the possibilities of students being matched with teachers across or beyond the divides of physical constraints (Wulf, 1993). Agre (2000) is critical of using the term 'revolutionary' and says, '... by caricaturing the old and idealizing the new, they falsely posit an absolute discontinuity between the past and the future'. However, within MDV education the opportunities for distance learning are great for postgraduates where the mores, values and workings of the profession are known. In fact, because of the distribution of practitioners a VLE may be the only method practicable.

Virtual learning alone is limited in undergraduate education where physical contact and involvement in the community of health workers is essential (see Chapter 8). Information technology should ideally be used as a means to amplify existing forces, and help make communication within the community more effective. Jill will be able to search for information quickly and send this by e-mail to Jack after their discussions. Jack can then start to formulate his questions about the lecture and e-mail these to the lecturer for clarification.

Problem-based learning (PBL)

Traditional MDV education would entail much discipline-based didactic teaching of pre-clinical knowledge to be followed separately by clinical practice. The students are largely left to themselves to integrate the two approaches. A full commitment to integration can be achieved by problem-based learning. The disciplines can then become seamless to the students, as they develop questions and learning objectives from case scenarios alone. The tutor shows the problem to the student group, without any suggested objectives. The group is then able to brainstorm the problem using standard procedures, of identifying unknown terminology, stating the issues involved, deducing hypotheses and finally formulating learning objectives. Following this meeting the students carry out self-directed learning. On a later occasion, the students then meet to present their findings, and in a cooperative way confirm, discuss and critically evaluate the information they have retrieved.

Problem-based learning as defined by Mayberry *et al* (1993) delivers a curriculum through a series of healthcare problems, discussed in a series of small group tutorial seminars, utilizing a student-centred approach to attain self-directed learning. This methodology has been strongly advocated for use in higher education (Wilkerson and Feletti, 1989) including medicine (Albanese and Mitchell, 1993) in dentistry (Ferrier 1990) and also in veterinary medicine (Rand and Baglioni, 1997).

Advantages and disadvantages of problem-based learning

Norman and Schmidt (1992) have indicated several potential advantages for students' learning claimed for problem-based learning. Students in PBL curricula may be more highly motivated; they may be better problem-solvers and self-directed learners; they may be better able to learn and recall information; and they may be better able to integrate basic science knowledge into the solutions of clinical problems. Barrows (1986) has schematized these points into:

- structuring knowledge for use in Clinical Contexts (SCC);
- developing an effective Clinical Reasoning Process (CRP);
- development of effective Self-Directed Learning skills (SDL);
- increased MOTivation for learning (MOT);

as if they were separate products that could be produced in the students. Meta-analysis-type reviews of medical undergraduate education over a period of 20 years (Albanese and Mitchell 1993;Vernon and Blake, 1993 and confirmed more recently by Colliver, 2000) have suggested that when compared with conventional instruction, PBL is more nurturing and enjoyable; PBL graduates perform as well, and sometimes better, on clinical examinations and faculty evaluations; and they are more likely to enter family medicine.

An articulate review paper on problem-based learning in dentistry is by Mayberry *et al* (1993) who strongly advocate a PBL approach. They favour this system because of the direct focus on objectives, the emphasis on student responsibility for self-directed learning, and small group peer support and feedback. They recommended the method especially at an introductory level for immersing the students into the cognitive aspects of the subject matter.

However, some authors have concerns about PBL. Ferrier (1990) writes, 'PBL gives students burdensome responsibilities for their own learning. What and how much they must study may no longer be clear'. More reservations from Albanese and Mitchell (1993) concern the kinds of backward thinking PBL graduates tended to use and possible gaps in their cognitive knowledge base that could affect practice outcomes. Patel, Groen and Norman (1991) also explain that when medical students are well grounded in the subject and are becoming more fluid in treatment planning difficult cases, they should be encouraged to practice 'expert' or 'forward reasoning', where it is possible to draw conclusions from highly selected but rather a small number of pieces of information. This contrasts with the alternative hypothetico-deductive PBL approach, so useful at the early stages of learning of the subject, but which may later tend to slow down thinking processes by producing extensive elaborations that generate errors.

Probably the most critical investigation of PBL is that by Fenwick and Parsons (1997) who find it offensive as practised, because they suggest that the highly selected 'cases' do not authentically represent human experience and perpetuate elitism by allowing professionals to construct an imaginary world for their students. They campaign for student interactions with patients in practice where attention is given to their overall well-being of the patient without necessarily the continual pressure to find productive solutions.

Straightforward practical difficulties have also been reported by Fincham *et al* (1997), who say that 'Pitfalls [in the PBL system]... include: weaker students being allocated less challenging issues; dominant students taking on their preferred tasks; and a failure to allocate key issues for research by all members of the group'. They add, 'Experience has shown that after a while a [PBL] group develops habits in that particular individuals will tend to take on repetitive roles as presenters or researchers. This can result in a staleness that can hamper the overall effectiveness of the group'.

Clearly, it is only when problem-based learning is used alone that it develops this other-worldliness. Unless the tutor system is highly developed in the small groups to give individual support, the total PBL curricula tend to be very centralized and standardized in organization, which focusses on the completion of learning blocks, problem outcomes and group functioning rather than individual development and practice. There is evidence that PBL is a challenging and active method that can be enjoyable, but there is less evidence for this to be the sole methodology. Albanese's (2000) excuse is that where there are mixed course 'Jurassic' didactic courses running concurrently that include tests and assignments, these will often force students to forgo a PBL course running parallel with it. Clearly there is a need for appropriate times allocated for self-directed learning and a balance of appropriate assessments in any curriculum, mono or mixed.

Problem-based learning has a place in the all-stakeholders curriculum. Used as a simulation method, early in the course, students like Jack will be delighted they are able to take a look at clinical cases as learning tools. In a protected learning environment he will find that he is given reserved time to research and draw from a number of hard copy and virtual sources seamlessly across disciplines. At a later time in the course, within a clinical speciality, for example, PBL can still be used as part of a teaching programme. It can be used as a means to ensure that Jill has knowledge of a certain range of conditions, by studying carefully chosen and ordered hypothetical clinical cases. By assuring standards the method may link well with concepts of competency that follow.

Influences of external agencies

There are various external agencies that would wish to influence the curriculum in MDV education. Most may have the aim to improve patient care and others to improve fairness in society. There are currently political pressures to increase the cultural diversity of students entering higher education (eg, CIHE, 2002). This is particularly a challenge in MDV education where standards and fitness for practice are closely associated with the cultural norms of the professions. Ways to widen access for students from disadvantaged areas are mentioned in Chapter 9 on supporting students. Draft MDV benchmarks have been issued by the Quality Assurance Authority (QAA, 2001) and are conservative estimates of standards against which curricula from different schools can be measured (Jackson and Lund, 2000). The value of benchmarks for educational courses is that they are agreed elements of content and process by experts in the field and can be used by teachers to assure themselves that core components in their courses comply. However, they have limited use in enhancing standards, unless they are 'stretch benchmarks', more commonly used in service industries, which include elements to which one could aspire, and plan to reach (Park City Solutions, 2001).

Curriculum stated in terms of outcomes or competency

Mager (1984) sets out the classic mode of organizing teaching in terms of general aims and in addition more specific objectives, which clearly describe the new behaviours the students are expected to learn, to what degree and in what context this can occur. More recently, educational programmes have been organized along 'learning outcomes'. These are items that are predetermined by the teacher, which indicate what the students will have learnt by the time they finish the course or module of learning. Quite a number of learning tasks undertaken in MDV clinical work appear at first sight to be merely procedural, and are skills that can and must be learnt, such as taking a blood sample or giving a local analgesic.

One way to clarify the learning outcomes required of students is to set out core competency statements (Hendricson and Kleffner, 1998). This involves the use of a set of minimum requirements for skills and knowledge to a particular standard that the students must reach by the time they qualify. This is useful for the student in a number of ways. The core compulsory knowledge and skills can be kept to manageable levels, and what is needed is made clear. When students are assessed, the requirements are criterion-based and not related to the relative abilities within a group of students. There can be time set aside for optional courses in subjects that particularly interest certain students, which can facilitate movement into a specialist area at a later date.

When it comes to teaching, efforts are concentrated on ensuring that the entire class pass, by reaching the standard required. This provides an opportunity to help create a climate for the student where the focus is on the collaborative working within the group, rather than individuals working in competition with each other (Kleffner and Dadian, 1997). If Jill is struggling in one particular core course, the group will function at a speed and in collaboration with each other to ensure that she has the minimum knowledge and skills demanded in the learning outcomes. In addition, a competency-based curriculum may make demands for staff to work together from different disciplines (Hendricson and Kleffner, 1998).

However, Stenhouse (1975), Bull (1985), Marshall (1991) and Callender (1992) have been particularly critical of attempts to place all aspects of a curriculum in competency format. They are concerned that a dogma will be created encouraging all aspects of practice outcome to be analysed, and progressively broken down into sub-competencies so that numbers of times a sub-competency has been reached can be slavishly recorded as a quota assessment. Stenhouse readily admits that the concepts of competencies may be useful at the early stages of an educational programme, but strongly asserts, 'knowledge is primarily concerned with synthesis. The analytic approach implied in the objectives model readily trivializes it... the best means of development is not by clarifying ends but by criticizing practice'.

Fortunately a number of authors who have recently embraced competency have done so as part of an educational process, not as an end in itself. For instance, Knox (1986) and Chambers and Gerrow (1994) see competency as a stage in the process of lifelong learning. The beginner soon becomes a novice in the profession, but it is only when they reach the prescribed standards that they can be deemed competent. After working and continuing learning for a number of years the MDV professional can become proficient and with adequate continuing professional development and experience, can reach mastery, the level of experts.

Excellence and competency – are they compatible?

In university mission statements there is often reference to excellence rather than competence. Are the two concepts compatible? As Elton (1996) says, most ideas of excellence come from the need for research to exceed current boundaries of knowledge to be worthy of reward. On the other hand everyone has to be taught and it is then more important to avoid incompetence than to have excellence. However, if the major competency statements of minimal levels of skills knowledge and attitudes, are enforced, but left sufficiently 'open-ended' to actively encourage those standards to be exceeded, criteria for excellence may have been reached (ie, highly competent; reflective; innovative; reaching more dimensions than competence [Elton, 1996]). However, when dealing with people, patients as well as other healthcare workers, 'how things are done' may be as important as the fact that they 'are done' at all (King, 1979). Perhaps the raw competencies alone as functions of 'knowledge, skills and standards' described by Kirschner *et al* (1997) are missing the attitudinal, affective elements that are essential for a new professional.

Barnett (1994) criticizes the simple acceptance of what he called operational competence, making students obey 'standards' of external competences derived from the world of work. He sees this as the creation of empty vessels that unthinkingly perform predetermined activities like automata. He emphasizes instead that education should entail a task of fulfilling internal demands for students to flourish and free themselves from the constraints under which they are already thinking and acting. This is a return to the primary consideration of the student, with a life story, moving and communicating, learning and developing appropriate skills in their work and internal resources to not only cope with change but to embrace it and work as agents of change.

Rather than a simplistic role for the MDV professional as a deliverer of services we require now, there should be a focus on the future in preparation for uncertainty. To prepare for this he suggests a greater need for reflection, dialogue, critique, development of consensus and practical understanding, as opposed to an emphasis on strategic outcomes.

Brew (1999) worries that an emphasis on having skills or being competent may serve to obscure important issues such as willingness to use that skill in a particular circumstance or judgement on when it is appropriate to use that skill. For instance, Jack may have the skills to take blood, but is he willing to perform this skill on a high-risk patient? Should Jill take the blood immediately following a glucose injection or after the patient has fasted? Brew sees the danger that competency-based curricula could lock students into a time warp. She sees self-assessment as an important means to allow students to evaluate and reject those competences that are no longer applicable.

Bowden and Marton (1998) also want to break away from the sense of competence meaning independent observable units of behaviour in the workplace. They wish to use the term in another way as capabilities of seeing and handling novel situations in powerful ways that integrate disciplinary and professional knowledge. In keeping with this view, when a clinician teaches Jack in a specialist clinic, one aim is for him to be able to focus critically on what he is doing and 'see things' from the specialist clinical point of view – to increase his repertoire of such views. His specific skills of taking a detailed history, observation, patient communication, investigations and treatment serve as adjunctive skills and are applied if and when required.

Conclusion

Bowden and Marton (1998) have shown that students need to experience a great deal of variation within a theme of skills that emphasize both relatedness and differences and to develop scenarios that work and do not work to learn and become adaptable to future unknowns. Working with patients produces an infinite range of variation that should be brought into the learning environment wherever possible. The use of variation can be taken one step further when considering curriculum design, which focusses on the student's 'way of seeing'. Following Bowden and Marton, it is suggested here that curriculum development should begin with an understanding of students like Jack and Jill. The principles of their learning should be analysed and the kind of learning environment that would suit them should be determined. It is important then for the curriculum developer to be open to a consideration of the range of learning experience that will assist students most, rather than finding the most convenient way for the teacher to deliver. If the curriculum based on learning outcomes of competences as 'core' external standards make Jack and Jill successful professionals today, the development of their critical thinking and inner skills of reflection and self-directed learning may be just as important as professionals working in an uncertain future.

References

Agre, P E (2000) Infrastructure and Institutional Change in the Networked University, *Information, Communication, and Society*, **3** (4), pp 494–507

Albanese, M A and Mitchell, S (1993) Problem-based learning: A Review of literature on its outcomes and implementation issues, [published erratum appears in *Academic Medicine*, 1993 Aug, **68** (8), p 615], *Academic Medicine*, 68 (1), pp 52–81

Albanese, M A (2000) Problem-based learning: why curricula are likely to show little effect on knowledge and clinical skills, *Medical Education*, **34**, pp 729–38

Barnett, R (1994) *The Limits of Competence*, The Society for Research into Higher Education and Open University Press, London

Barrows, H S (1986) A taxonomy of problem-based learning methods, *Medical Education*, **20**, pp 481–86

Bertolami, C N (2001) Rationalizing the Dental Curriculum in Light of Current Disease Prevalence and Patient Demand for Treatment: Form vc, Content, *Journal of Dental Education*, **65** (8), pp 725–35

Bowden, J and Marton, F (1998) *The University of Learning*, Kogan Page, London

Brew, A (1999) Towards Autonomous Assessment: Using Self-Assessment and Peer Assessment, in *Assessment Matters in Higher Education: Choosing and Using Diverse Approaches*, eds S Brown and A Glaser, pp 159–71, SRHE, London

Brown, G and Atkins, M (1997) Explaining, in *The Handbook of Communication Skills*, ed O D W Hargie, 2nd edn, pp 183–212, Routledge, London

Bruffee, K A (1993) *Collaborative Learning: Higher Education, Interdependence, and the Authority of Knowledge*, paperback edn 1995, The John Hopkins University Press, Baltimore and London

Bull, H (1985) The Use of Behavioural Objectives, *Journal of Further and Higher Education*, **9** (1), pp 74–80

Callender, C (1992) *Will NVQs Work? Evidence from the Construction Industry*, University of Sussex/Institute of Manpower Studies, Sussex

Chambers, D W and Gerrow, J D (1994) Manual for Developing and Formatting Competency Statements, *Journal of Dental Education*, **58**, pp 559–64

CIHE (2002) Encouraging Learning and Excellence through a Sustained Partnership, *The Council for Industry and Higher Education* [Online] http://www.cihe-uk.com/http://www.cihe-uk.com/

Coles, C R (1977) *Curriculum Evaluation: The Southampton Perspective*, paper presented at ASME/SRHE Conference, 30th November

Colliver, J (2000) Effectiveness of problem based learning curricula, *Academic Medicine*, **75**, pp 259–66

Delanty, G (2001) *Challenging Knowledge: The University in the Knowledge Society*, SRHE and OUP, London

Elton, L (1996) Criteria for Teaching Competence and Teaching Excellence in Higher Education, in *Evaluating Teacher Quality in Higher Education*, eds R Aylett and K Gregory, pp 33–41, Falmer, London

Fenwick, T J and Parsons, J (1997) *A Critical Investigation of the Problems with Problem-Based Learning*, Eric document ED 409272

Ferrier, B M (1990) Problem-based Learning: Does it Make a Difference, *Journal of Dental Education*, **54**, pp 550–51

Fincham A G *et al* (1997) Problem-based Learning at the University of Southern California School of Dentistry, *Journal of Dental Education*, **61**, pp 417–25

Genn, J M (2001) AMEE Medical Education Guide No 23 (Part 1): Curriculum, environment, climate, quality and change in medical education – a unifying perspective, *Medical Teacher*, **23**, pp 337–44

GMC (1993) *Tomorrow's Doctors: Recommendations on Undergraduate Medical Education* [Online] http://www.gmc-uk.org/meded/*meded*frameset.htm http://www.gmc-uk.org/meded/*meded*frameset.htm

Habermas, J (1991) *The New Conservatism: Cultural Criticism and the Historians' Debate*, MIT Press, Cambridge, MA

Harden, R M (2001) The learning environment and the curriculum, *Medical Teacher*, **23**, pp 335–36

Harden, R M, Sowden, S, and Dunn, W R (1984) *Some Educational Strategies in Curriculum Development: The SPICES Model*, Medical Education Booklet edn v 18, ASME, Edinburgh

Hendricson, W D and Kleffner, J H (1998) Curricular and Instructional Implications of Competency-Based Dental Education, *Journal of Dental Education*, **62**, pp 183–96

Jackson, N and Lund, H (2000) *Benchmarking for Higher Education*, SRHE and OUP, Buckingham

Kern, D E, Thomas, P A, and Howard, D M *et al* (1998) *Curriculum Development For Medical Education, A Six Step Approach*, John Hopkins University Press, Baltimore and London

Kerr, J F (1968) *Changing the Curriculum*, University of London Press, London

King, S (1979) Assessment of Competence: Technical Problems and Publications, in *On Competence: A Critical Analysis of Competence-Based Reforms in Higher Education*, ed G Grant, 1st edn, pp 491–520, Jossey-Bass, San Francisco

Kirschner, P, Van Vilsteren, P and Hummel, H *et al* (1997) The Design of a Study Environment for Acquiring Academic and Professional Competence, *Studies in Higher Education*, **22**, pp 151–71

Kleffner, J H and Dadian, T (1997) Using Collaborative Learning in Dental Education, *Journal of Dental Education*, **61**, pp 66–72

Knox, A B (1986) *Helping Adults Learn: A Guide to Planning, Implementing, and Conducting Programs*, Jossey-Bass, San Francisco

Kolb, D A (1984) *Experiential learning experience as the source of learning and development*, Prentice-Hall, Englewood Cliffs

Mager, R F (1984) *Preparing Instructional Objectives*, revised 2nd edn, David S Lake, Belmont, California

Marshall, K (1991) NVQs: An assessment of the 'Outcomes' Approach in Education and Training, *Journal of Further and Higher Education*, **16** (2), pp 71–79

Mayberry, W E *et al* (1993) *An Introduction to Problem-Based Learning*, University Missouri-Kansas

Norman, G R and Schmidt, H G (1992) The psychological basis of problem-based learning: a review of the evidence [Review], *Academic Medicine*, **67** (9), pp 557–65

Park City Solutions (2001) *Benchmarking – Introduction* [Online] http://www.pcslabservices.com/introduction.htm

Patel, V L, Groen, G J and Norman, G R (1991) Effects of conventional and problem-based medical curricula on problem solving, *Academic Medicine*, **66** (7), pp 380–89

QAA (2001) *Dentistry – Academic Standards* [Online] http–www.qaa.ac.uk-crntwork-benchmark-phase2-dentistry.pdf

Rand, J S and Baglioni, A J (1997) Subject-based problem-based learning in the Veterinary Science course at the University of Queensland, *Australian Veterinary Journal*, **75**, pp 120–25

Randall, F and Downie, R S (1999) *Palliative Care Ethics: A Companion for all Specialties*, 2nd edn, OUP, Oxford

Socket, H (1976) *Designing the Curriculum*, Open Books, London

Stenhouse, L (1975) *An Introduction to Curriculum Research and Development*, Heinemann Educational Books, London

Vernon, D T and Blake, R L (1993) Does problem-based learning work? A meta-analysis of evaluative research [see comments], *Academic Medicine*, **68** (7), pp 550–63

Wilkerson, L A and Feletti, G (1989) Problem-Based Learning: One Approach to Increasing Student Participation, *New Directions for Teaching and Learning*, **37**, pp 51–60

Wulf, W A (1993) The collaboratory opportunity, *Science*, 13 August, pp 854–55

5

Assessment of the student practitioner

Joy Crosby

Introduction

Assessment is perhaps one of the most important aspects of a student's higher educational experience. This chapter covers the role of assessment, the principles of assessment, tools of assessment, who should assess, when should assessment take place and the importance of evaluating the assessment process.

The role of assessment

A recent edition of the *British Medical Journal* (*BMJ*) highlighted an excerpt from the journal in 1901 (*BMJ*, 2001):

> But there are three things which you must learn in your five years of medical study. You have to learn how to learn. Then you have to learn as much as you can of those things which are of immediate and cardinal importance, and which will serve as the groundwork for future learning after you commence practice. Lastly, you have to learn how to set forth what you have learned in such a manner as to persuade a Board of Examiners that you are fit and proper persons to be let loose on the public as qualified medical practitioners.

This quote demonstrates how little medical education has changed in the last 100 years. More importantly the quote makes explicit the function of assessment in its most accepted and public sense, that of judging fitness to practice, but also highlights two areas of the learning process – personal self-development and promulgation of knowledge through teaching – which can also be informal and shaped by assessment. The effectiveness of assessment depends on the reasons for its use, which may vary in importance. These reasons have been grouped into four key areas:

- the promotion of student development;
- to inform teaching;
- to identify quality;
- to make judgements.

Features of assessment

Assessment motivates a student to learn (Brown and Knight, 1994). However, motivation to succeed may result in heightened anxiety that obscures the true abilities of an individual. Timely feedback from assessment is fundamental to learning (Rowntree, 1987) and can serve to identify a student's strengths and weaknesses. The ability to assess one's own competence, as well as that of others, is crucial to lifelong learning. Assessment may encourage students to focus either more on independent revision or the setting up of study groups. Members of staff may wish to assess students to find out how effectively they (the staff) have facilitated learning. The quality of teaching may influence the learning acquired. Performance in assessment may be indicative of this learning. This may have obvious implications for the teaching programme where poor student performance may identify deficits in the learning programme and provide feedback for curriculum planners and teachers.

One of the most important functions of assessment is to satisfy external bodies that students are competent to practice. A school has a responsibility to ensure that only competent students progress through the course. There is also a place for recognition of excellence and the allocation of prizes. An assessment that records how a student excels may help a student's future career progression.

Principles of assessment

Several principles can be used to guide assessment:

1. **Assessment should respond to the learning programme**
   Students as strategic individuals work on what will be assessed; 'assessment drives the curriculum'. But care has to be taken by curriculum planners that it does not drive the planning of the curriculum. It is important that outcomes specified by a school should dictate what is assessed and what the students are expected to learn.
2. **Formative and summative assessments should be used**
   Summative assessment is used 'to decide' and formative 'to improve' (Scrivens, 1967). Summative assessment is that which 'sums up someone's achievement

and which has no other real use except as a description of what has been achieved' (Brown and Knight, 1994). Formative assessment is that which informs students of their knowledge or performance, and is dependent upon the quality of the feedback given. Unfortunately this may incur a large additional workload to those concerned (Rolfe and McPherson, 1995). However, formative assessments may have the advantage that they encourage students to adopt deeper approaches to learning (Entwistle, 1992; see Chapter 7 of this book).

3. **A range of valid, reliable, feasible and authentic tools of assessment should be used**

A mixed economy of methods should be adopted in order that the multidimensional nature of learning can be adequately assessed. The assessment tools used must be valid, reliable, feasible and authentically represent the situation in which the learning will be used.

A **valid** assessment should assess what is to be measured (Brown, Race and Smith, 1996). A valid assessment will permit conclusions to be drawn about the ability of a student (see recommended reading list below).

Reliable refers to a consistency of assessment results (Grounlund and Linn, 1985). Individuals must be able to answer a question in the same way on two different occasions. In addition, examiners should also be reliable. Intra-tester reliability determines that an examiner will come to the same grade on two separate occasions when marking the same piece of work. This can be achieved with the help of clear marking schemes and paying attention to fatigue that could influence marking performance. Many examinations use a second marker. Inter-tester reliability is achieved when a number of examiners are able to reach the same grade when marking the same piece of work (see recommended reading list).

Authentic relates to the realism of the assessment (Torrance, 1995). For example, in assessing a student's ability to take blood pressure, low authenticity may be indicated for a test on a simulator in a laboratory, moderate authenticity for a peer or simulated patient and high authenticity for a real patient in the clinical setting.

Limited numbers of trained staff and resources to set up, run, mark and deliver feedback to students may prevent some institutions from attempting an assessment protocol. Overall, a high level of validity, reliability, feasibility, and authenticity may not be possible in some assessments, which may still be considered worthwhile. For example, assessing performance while in a workplace situation may be valid but establishing reliability may be problematic. The opposite is also true. It is possible to establish a high reliability in formal exams but validity for professional development may be questioned. Similarly a useful authentic assessment may pose real problems in terms of **feasibility**. Table 5.1 shows a matrix of the four issues against commonly used tools of assessment.

Table 5.1 Assessment methods

	Validity	**Reliability**	**Feasibility**	**Effect on Learning**
Method	what is being measured?	would the same result be obtained if the assessment was repeated?	are the resources and time available to run the assessment?	how will the assessment affect student behaviour?
MCQ	recognition of facts if negatively marked exam technique and risk-taking	good reliability objective scoring	quick and cheap	surface approach is encouraged reliance on books
OSCE	clinical skills	checklists and global rating scales may be used case specificity	labour intensive for the duration of the assessment	encyclopaedic approach practical experience valued
Triple Jump	problem-solving and research skills ability to orally present in a logical manner	poor reliability different for each candidate	labour intensive although may be spread over a period of time	emphasis on clinical/ academic work may seek out patients
Essays	knowledge and understanding of a topic ability to express in the written form scores affected by writing skills may not relate to practice	marking criteria required without criteria poor subjective marking	labour intensive although often throughout the year	encourages logical note-taking, practical clinical work may not be necessary
Portfolio	evidence of learning performance may be affected by presentation skills	clear criteria required depends on how extensive the range of the portfolio material	labour-intensive marking takes time	may encourage reflection and continuous work
Observational On-the-job	clinical skills, attitudes, application of knowledge face validity for on-the-job skills	interreliability may be poor objectivity questionable without checklists	should be embedded within the job	emphasis on importance of day-to-day activities

4. **Standards should be set**
Traditionally three types of standard setting can be considered:
- criteria referenced;
- norm referenced;
- personal referenced.

Standard determined by criteria
The use of criterion referencing is common in MDV education where students have to meet certain criteria in order to 'pass'. One of the most widely used methods for setting the standard is the modified Angoff (Friedman Ben-David, 2000). A 'pass' mark is based on the decision of a panel of persons reflecting on the performance they consider acceptable. The 'pass mark' and the associated criteria are made explicit both to staff and students prior to the examination sitting.

Standard determined by the norm
Normative standard setting looks at the norm distribution of results. Historically, a bell-shaped curve has represented this distribution with the majority of students receiving marks within the body of the bell and the trailing edges representing the few students with low scores on one side and high scores on the other.

The grades are referenced by the average, norm score, and therefore may vary from exam to exam and from student group or year. The standard is how the student relates to others in the class. The disadvantage of this method is that it has the potential of indicating that weak students should pass if the average score in that instance was poor.

Standard determined by personal performance
The term 'personal standard' assessment has been coined here to indicate that individuals respond to their own standard, attempting to improve on standards they have previously set (Brown and Knight, 1994). These methods have potential in MDV education with the current emphasis on personal development and self-assessment. Each method of setting the standard has its own merits and are summarized in Table 5.2.

Table 5.2 Type of referencing and when to use it

Types of Referencing	Examples of When to Use
Criterion	assessment of competence utilized for core assessments where all student should reached a prescribed level of competence standard setting process should be used – eg, Angoff
Normative	assessment by comparing with the norm, useful for the placing of students may be used for elective, special study modules and prizes to differentiate students
Personal	focus on the improvement of the individual may be used within part of a portfolio assessment

5. **Feedback should be given to students**
   Feedback is only important if assessment is seen to have a role in facilitating learning. Feedback is perhaps the single most important factor related to learning (Rowntree, 1987) and may be maximized if it is:
   - provided frequently;
   - given in a timely manner;
   - given under stress-free conditions;
   - meaningful (Rolfe and McPherson, 1995).

   Immediacy places pressure on the staff to respond within a given time frame. Constructive feedback given in a timely manner is sometimes difficult to achieve due to a large number of students. Students need an explanation for what is not up to standard, and more importantly, what is the correct standard. Computer-assisted packages may be utilized to give feedback especially where the responses are quite limited, for example in MCQs (multiple-choice questions) or short answer responses.
6. **Assessment should be transparent to students**
   Assessment should be seen as a helpful aid to learning and not to catch students out (Harden, 1979). Students need to know at the beginning of their course of study what they may be assessed on, the criteria used to assess, the standard expected and the consequences should they fail.
7. **The effect on learning should be considered and evaluated**
   Assessment affects what and how a student learns (Newble and Jaeger, 1983). If assessment is mainly practically based, then students will attempt to seek out patients and develop competence in skills. If assessment requires rote learning, then the effect on learning will be to study lecture notes and information in books. The content of assessment will also influence what the student learns.
8. **Support should be given to failing students**
   Assessment can be stressful. Failure in assessment may have serious implications for a student. Support should be given to help students remediate or acknowledge deficits that result in termination of studies.

Tools of assessment

For the purpose of this section assessment methods have been separated into areas that focus on recall of knowledge, problem-solving skills, practical skills, group work, personal goals and the holistic learner.

Focus on recall of knowledge

Knowledge is an important aspect of clinical practice and can be tested by asking students to choose the correct answer from a range of responses – commonly known as multiple-choice questions (MCQs).The following are some examples of commonly used techniques.

True/false

The student has to make a judgement whether each statement is true or false. All, none or some of the statements may be true. For example (Harding Rains, 1996):

The symptoms of cellulitis include:
A pain
B throbbing
C the presence or absence of pulsation
D ballottement
E emptying and filling

The student has a 50 per cent chance of guessing correctly.

Matching items and extended matching items

In matching items the student is expect to choose the right answer out of a series of responses. If five responses are given there is a 20 per cent chance of guessing the right answer. In recent years 'extended matching items' (EMIs) have been developed where the number of potential answers is increased. For example:

The patient has developed endocarditis, has not received any antibiotic therapy and blood cultures are all regular. What is the most likely infecting organism?

A Staphylococcus epidermis	F Staphylococcus aureus
B Klebsiella pneumoniae	G Enterococcus pneumoniae
C Candida albicans	H Streptococcus pneumoniae
D Escherichia coli	I Enterococcus faecalis
E Streptococcus 'viridans'	J Coxiella burnetii

Extended matching items attempt to reduce the chance element by increasing the number of choices available to the student. In this way if 10 options are given rather than two, as in true or false questions, the likelihood of guessing is reduced from 50 per cent to 10 per cent.

There has been much criticism regarding the MCQ type of questions. Research suggests that students may be cued into a superficial approach to learning and select answers with little understanding. Guessing the right response may be used to some effect with true/false questions. In order to combat this, negative marking can be used, which penalizes the student by subtracting a mark when an incorrect answer is given. This can result in the student receiving a sub zero mark. Unfortunately, students find negative marking extremely stressful and test results may indicate a student's risk-taking attitude (Premadasa, 1993) or examination technique (Hammond *et al*, 1998) rather than knowledge. Generating appropriate

MCQs is also time-consuming and difficult. However, well-designed questions could provide benefits, especially where the distracter responses (the 'wrong' ones) represent common student misconceptions and where they could be used in computer-assisted learning (CAL) packages (Khan, Davies and Gupta, 2001).

Short answers

Short answer questions are being more widely used. The following are examples of such questions.

1. Arterial blood pressure is the product of cardiac output and ______________
2. A patient presents with thirst and headaches. What investigations would you suggest? ____

Whilst the above questions are self-contained, short answers may be constructed to evolve in an attempt to replicate practice. Short answer questions reduce the amount of potential cuing seen in MCQs. Care must be taken to ensure that students are able to complete all parts of the questions and are not blocked by an incorrect response during an early part of the questions. Such questions can have high validity and allow concepts to be tested using real-life examples. One of the main drawbacks of short answer questions is that all of them must be judged and marked. This may become an administrative job if the possible correct answers are clearly defined but marking can be a time-consuming process.

Essay types

Essay questions may attempt to assess many aspects of learning. They may be used to demonstrate a student's ability to reason coherently; to show an understanding of a topic. The essay can capture the capacity of the student to use high-level intellectual skills to consider complex issues from a range of perspectives. However, an essay fails to capture the authentic environment of the clinical world. Its reliability is questionable without clear, objective marking criteria. Criteria should include model answers with a description of what is required with marks assigned. They can potentially help examiners save time marking and can also increase the reliability of the assessors (Brown, Race and Smith, 1996). One potential downside of the essay as a tool of assessment is the opportunity for plagiarism. Whilst there are computer packages to spot plagiarism, some may be averted by ensuring that students have clear guidelines regarding correct use and referencing of other authors' material (Rennie and Crosby, 2002).

Long case

In a typical long case a student spends an hour with a patient then is orally examined. Gleeson (1997) attempted to improve the validity and reliability of the long case by developing the objective structured long examination record

(OSLER) introducing a prescribed 10-item analysis. The OSLER also allows the difficulty of the case to be taken into account (see recommended reading).

Problem-solving skills – triple jump

The triple jump is an assessment method that was devised to assess a student's ability at considering a clinical problem within the problem-based learning environment (Smith, 1993). It mirrors the problem-based learning cycle (see Chapter 7 later in this book). The three stages to the triple jump are as follows:

- Stage 1 The assessor presents the student with a clinical problem. From this the student generates key learning issues.
- Stage 2 The student researches the learning issues identified in Stage 1.
- Stage 3 The student returns to the assessor and discusses the case.

This type of assessment has the potential of accurately mimicking clinical practice. It focusses on the process of learning and the ability to identify learning issues and address them. The triple jump can be both an authentic and valid form of assessment. Drawbacks are that it is manpower-intensive and the subjective nature of the assessment could lead to lack of reliability. Resources must be available for students in order to answer issues identified. However, there is scope for integrating self- and peer assessment within this assessment method to improve reliability.

Focus on practical and clinical skills

Assessments that reflect the work of the clinical practitioner are a challenge in MDV education (Mavis, Cole and Hoppe, 2001). Currently, the objective structured clinical examination (OSCE) is the most widely used assessment of clinical performance (Harden and Gleeson, 1979).

Objective structured clinical examination (OSCE)

The OSCE requires the student to complete a task in a designated period of time in a controlled, often simulated environment. Invariably an OSCE has a number of stations (between 20 and 40) between which the student rotates, completing a variety of tasks. Many of the stations will utilize patients, or simulated patients, and require an examiner to mark the student completing the task. The examiner uses a checklist in order to make the assessment objective. Table 5.3 shows an example of one station in an OSCE. The example includes the instructions the student is given, the resources required to run the station and the checklist. The drawbacks of the OSCE are the extensive demands on resources.

Table 5.3 OSCE

Student instructions: At this station please take the patient's blood pressure.
Resources required: Patient or simulated patient, manual manometer, stethoscope.
Instructions to examiner: Ask the student to take the patient's blood pressure. Using the checklist record the student's performance.
Blood pressure checklist:
Tick 0 if not performed inadequately
Tick 1 if adequately performed

Blood Pressure	Mark	
	0	1
Explain the procedure to the patient		
• particularly that there may be discomfort when inflating the cuff		
• also that the measurement may be taken more than once		
Ensure the patient is lying/sitting on the bed/couch		
The arm should be horizontal and supported at the level of the mid-sternum		
Correctly position the cuff on the upper arm with the bladder positioned over the brachial artery		
Ensure the mercury column in the manometer is vertical		
Estimate the systolic pressure by palpating the brachial artery and inflating the cuff until the pulsation disappears		
Place the stethoscope over the brachial artery		
Inflate the cuff until pressure is 30 mmHg over the estimated systolic pressure		
Reduce the pressure at 2–3 mmHg/sec		
Auscultate the systolic pressure at which clear tapping sounds are heard		
Auscultate the diastolic pressure at the point where the sounds disappear		
Give the recording of the blood pressure to the nearest 2 mmHg		

Adapted from the recommendations of the British Hypertension Society

Observational techniques

Assessments based on direct observation in the clinical setting have been advocated by Cohen (2001). Without clear marking descriptors and consistent supervision this method of assessment is notoriously subjective and unreliable. However, the authenticity and feasibility of such an approach ensure that this is a useful assessment method. Observation of clinical skills can be on site or via video recording, which may allow closer critique in a less pressurized environment. The structured clinical operative test (SCOT) has been recently introduced (Mossey and Newton, 2001). A checklist similar to the OSCE is devised, which is transparent and accessible by both staff and students. It is used in the authentic clinical setting, for example, wards, clinics and operating theatres, and may have both a formative and summative role (Rennie and Crosby, 2002). Students in the first instance would be introduced in a supervised setting to the operative test with the checklist as a guide and then encouraged to use it for self- or peer assessment. When the student feels confident, a staff member may then assess the student summatively, although also giving formative feedback to the student.

Focus on personal skills

Increasingly, attention is being placed on the personal qualities of students. Personal qualities may include attitudes to patients, relatives or owners of animals, ability to be reflective and constructively critical, and the ability to take responsibility for own learning. Personal qualities are difficult to assess. Whilst the OSCE has been successfully utilized as an objective means of assessing interpersonal communication skills, observational techniques may be the most valid method of assessing other personal qualities but often these are unreliable. A devious individual may be able to mask inappropriate personal qualities during an examination period with those that seem appropriate. Although certain aspects of learning may be difficult to assess it is important not to restrict students' learning just to what can be easily assessed. The learning experience would be impoverished if this stance were taken.

A number of assessment forms have been devised to record the important issues of team working (see Table 5.4). Both tutors and peers should be involved in the assessment of group work, ensuring confidentiality where necessary. Determining individual contributions to group work is important and Conway *et al* (1993) devised a marking formula: individual student mark = individual weighting factor × final group project mark.

Table 5.4 Personal qualities

Mark the student by giving a mark of 1 to 5 in each of the following categories:

	5	4	3	2	1	
makes regular constructive contributions to the group						does not contribute constructively to the group
confident that work allocated will be completed appropriately						no confidence that the work allocated will be completed
works well with other members of the group						does not work well with other members of the group
is helpful and courteous						is unhelpful and rude
able to plan and prioritize tasks						not able to plan and prioritize tasks
able to organize and supervise others						not able to organize and supervise others
grasps essentials very quickly						very slow at recognizing essentials
anticipates the requirements of new situations and takes appropriate action						has difficulty in recognizing implications of new situation
is good at solving problems						not able to solve problems appropriately

Form modified from Robert Gordon University, School of Computer and Mathematical Science

The individual weighting factor was devised to address the unfairness of giving all students the same mark irrespective of their contribution (Cheng and Warren, 2000). It is calculated by dividing the individual effort rating by the average effort rating of the group. The individual effort rating can be calculated by summing the marks peer group members give a student on a variety of different parameters. The average rating of the group can be calculated by adding the individual ratings and dividing by the number of students in the group.

Focus on the holistic learner

A student in MDV practice will be expected to demonstrate appropriate personal attributes and utilize knowledge and practical skills together. Assessment strategies are available that attempt to assess the holistic learner.

Portfolio assessment

A portfolio is a collection of work that shows the student's learning over a period of time. It is the learner's responsibility to create, maintain and, when necessary, present the portfolio for assessment (Snadden, Thomas and Challis, 1999). The *Dearing Report* (1997) into higher education has recommended the use of portfolios in both undergraduate and postgraduate education. In medicine, the portfolio is a key feature of revalidation (GMC, 2000) as it provides evidence of lifelong learning, professional development and self-learning. The benefits of portfolio assessment include the emphasis on continuous assessment. The portfolio can offer a realistic representation of individuals' work over a period of time. In addition, a portfolio can offer a useful structure for learning and will facilitate development of skills of accountability for one's own learning. Portfolios may also offer an opportunity for students to demonstrate learning outcomes that may be difficult to assess in traditional types of assessment such as those related to attitudes and personal development. Portfolios at an undergraduate level will also give some experience to the learner in preparation for portfolio requirements in the postgraduate setting. The requirement to collect evidence of learning will begin to establish the skills of accountability for learning.

The major disadvantage of portfolio assessment is the administrative and staff workload required in assessing a portfolio. Students may regard portfolios as onerous/burdensome, something done by jumping through hoops. If students hold this attitude the projected advantages in terms of learning may not materialize. There are also concerns regarding the reliability of the use of portfolios as a method of assessment. The diverse, unique collection of work from a student makes the formulation of assessment criteria a challenge, but these can be refined as experience in their use is gained.

Who should assess?

In the past, the emphasis has been on the staff who assess students. This narrow perspective supposes that assessment is fundamentally to determine progression of a student. However, the ability to assess is a personal attribute that should be encouraged in the development of students.

Staff

Using staff has the advantage that they are: knowledgeable; appointed due to their expertise in a specific area; should not be biased; may be skilled in assessment; and are paid to perform the task. Assessment is a recognized role of the teacher (Harden and Crosby, 2001) and an important aspect of the professional teacher's duties.

Student self-assessment

Self-assessment is becoming more in vogue in higher education with the acceptance that it is a key tenet of adult learning (Brookfield, 1988). Lifelong learners are expected to continually assess themselves and will need to practice at undergraduate level. One of the concerns regarding self-assessment has been in questioning the accuracy of marking written papers. Research is inconclusive; some students giving lower marks, higher marks (Mahalski, 1992), and accurate marking (Falchikov and Boud, 1989). The best advice would be to pilot any initiative in self-marking. Approaches that may be used to promote self-assessment are commonly the completion of log books where students self-certify when they feel competent in a skill. Certain aspects of learning can only be self-assessed. For example, the confidence felt when completing a skill or procedure or the amount of effort allocated to a task.

Peer assessment

Peers have an invaluable role to play in some types of assessment. In dentistry it has been found that senior students can be used to accurately assess junior students in basic technical skills (Ogden, Green and Ker, 2000). Peer assessment of communication skills or team working may also be particularly useful. In assessing another student's written material or skills the student may develop a better grasp of the material (Falchikov, 1995). The process of assessing may improve the ability to give constructive criticism (Falchikov, 1995) and appreciation of the assessment process (Brindley and Scoffield, 1998).

For certain skills, peers may be the only cohorts who can assess another student's contribution to work produced by a small group. But not all topics may be suitable for peer assessment. Clearly, issues of loyalty, collusion or settling old scores must be avoided. As they assess, peers will be developing graduate skills of critical judgement and decision-making. Although low marker variability of written papers has been found with peer assessment (King, Gray and Hossacks, 1992) if good criteria are given, the student may lack a certain degree of sophistication in the ability to assess a topic or performance that is not straightforward.

Patients

In MDV, patients and their carers (or their owners in the case of animals) may play a significant role in assessing student performance. Patients can be invaluable assessors especially for formative assessment (see Chapter 3). Communication skills require the interaction with another person. This person is usually a patient, relative or colleague, or a simulated actor. Although an examiner may be assessing the technical precision of a communication episode it is difficult for them to assess aspects like empathy and clarity. The person involved in the interaction may best assess these.

When should assessment take place?

Assessment should take place in a timely manner and be embedded into the learning programme if it is to facilitate learning. If the assessment is to help students make choices then it needs to take place prior to the choices being made.

Continuous assessment

The use of assessment to progress students continues to be one of the main purposes of assessment. It has been recommended by the General Medical Council (GMC, 1993) and the General Dental Council (GDC, 1997) that all schools should move to a system of continuous assessment. The rationale for such a statement is that a traditional 'hurdle' examination may not necessarily reflect the learning of a student over a period of time. Continuous assessments of ongoing work through the production of log books and portfolios are becoming more popular. The regular use of 'hurdle' assessment does not seem to encapsulate the spirit of continuous assessment, although called 'continuous' by some.

End of year assessments

In clinical disciplines the 'big bang' end of year degree examinations have been common. End of year examinations tend to sample work covered over a long period of time. It seems unfair that the learning of an individual should be judged by performance at such a brief moment in time.

Long loop assessments

Long loop assessments include the assessment of material that will have been taught and/or assessed previously in the course. The intention with the long loop assessment is to ensure that students do not forget crucial material covered in previous elements of the course and to reduce the mentality of the student that once something is assessed it can be forgotten (see Figure 5.1). Long loops should include only core material, which requires utilization in later parts of the course.

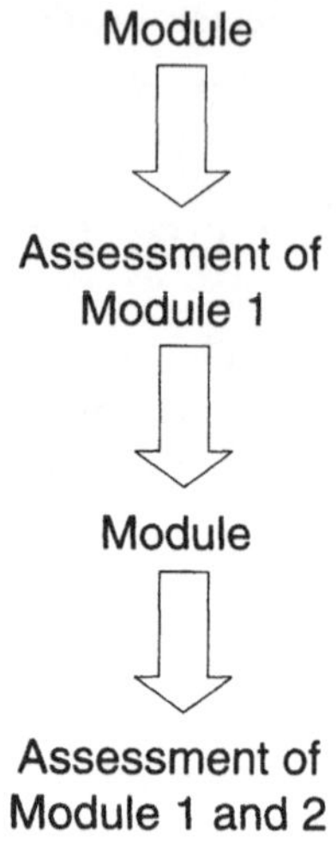

Figure 5.1 Long loop assessment

Progress test

A progress test is an assessment that is given to all years of the curriculum developed in PBL (problem-based learning) schools (van der Vleuten, Verwijnen and Wijnen, 1996). The level and content of the questions, although not the same questions, are the same for each year. The premise of the progress test is that as the student progresses through the course they achieve a higher proportion of correct results. It may be predicted that first-year students may, on average, correctly answer 20 per cent, second-year, 35 per cent and third-year, 50 per cent of the test questions. The progress tests to date tend to focus on the knowledge component of a course.

Evaluating the assessment process

A final aspect to consider is the importance of evaluating the assessment process. This is crucial as it provides a means to maintain quality and confidence in the assessment process. Aspects of assessment evaluation are outlined in Table 5.5 (adapted from Fowell, Southgate and Bligh, 1999). Evaluation should include the views of the students (especially level 3). Students may have legitimate views regarding the timing and running of the examination, the content and format, the value of feedback given and the effects of the assessment on their learning.

Table 5.5 Elements of the assessment process to be evaluated

Data	**Purpose**
Student performance per question – item (level 1 evaluation)	Determine student performance in an assessment and indirectly the teaching associated with the area of study. This data must be given to the relevant teachers delivering the course as well as the students.
Tests of reliability and validity of the test (level 2 evaluation)	Test of intra-tester and inter-tester reliability. Determine any reliability differences between markers, for example do content experts mark differently from non-content experts? Tests are very resource- and time-dependent. Correlation between tests may also be examined.
Running of the assessment (level 3 evaluation)	The process of planning the assessment, commissioning of questions, communication with students, running of the actual examinations and the presentation of results should all be evaluated. An external examiner may be helpful for all these elements.
Trends in assessment (level 4 evaluation)	Observation of general trends will be helpful in determining major changes in the assessment process. Data may have to be collected over a period of time to identify consistent trends, for example consistently poor performance by the majority of students in one aspect of the course, poor performance by an identifiable cohort of students, etc.

Levels 1 to 3 will offer immediate feedback regarding the assessment process whereas level 4 offers a more long-term view (Fowell *et al*, 1999).

Conclusion

Assessment is an important aspect of higher education. The purpose of assessment should determine the methods to be used and whether or not feedback is necessary. It is suggested that assessment has an important role in facilitating students' learning and that any school should include learning as one of their reasons for assessing students.

There are a variety of different tools available to assess students and a combination of these may best achieve the purpose of the assessment. The validity, reliability, authenticity and feasibility of any assessment tool should be considered.

Self- and peer assessment should be introduced as they have the potential of developing skills that will be important in the postgraduate setting and in lifelong learning. The process of assessment should be evaluated in order to ensure confidence in and the quality of the assessment process.

Assessment is important but should be put in context. The purpose of study in a degree in MDV is to produce competent independent practitioners. Assessment should aid that process and should not be seen in isolation from the importance of learning.

References

BMJ (2001) One hundred years ago: Perspectives in medical education, *British Medical Journal*, **322**, pp 958

Brindley, C and Scoffield, S (1998) Peer assessment in undergraduate programmes, *Teaching in Higher Education*, **3** (1), pp 78–89

Brookfield, S D (1988) *Understanding and facilitating adult learning*, OUP, Buckingham

Brown, S and Knight, P (1994) *Assessing Learners in Higher Education*, Kogan Page, London

Brown, S, Race, P and Smith, B (1996) *500 Tips on Assessment*, Kogan Page, London

Cheng, W and Warren, M (2000) Making a difference: using peers to assess individual students' contributions to a group project, *Teaching in Higher Education*, **5** (2), pp 243–55

Cohen, R (2001) Assessing professional behaviour and medical error, *Medical Teacher*, **23** (2), pp 145–51

Conway, R *et al* (1993) Peer assessment of an individual's contribution to a group project, *Assessment and Evaluation in Higher Education*, **18** (1), pp 45–56

Dearing, R (1997) *Report of the National Committee of Inquiry into Higher Education*, Chapter 9, p 20, [Online] http://www.leeds.ac.uk/educol/ncihe/

Entwistle, N (1992) Influences on the quality of student learning – implications for medical education, *South African Medical Journal*, **81**, pp 596–606

Falchikov, N and Boud, D (1989) Student self-assessment in higher education: a meta analysis, *Review of Educational Research*, **59** (4), pp 395–430

Falchikov, N (1995) Peer feedback marking: developing peer assessment, *Innovations in Education and Training International*, **32** (2), pp 175–87

Fowell, S I, Southgate, L J and Bligh, J G (1999) Evaluating assessment: the missing link, *Medical Education*, **33**, pp 276–81

Friedman Ben-David, M (2000) *Standard Setting in Student Assessment*, AMEE Medical Education Guide No 18, Dundee, Scotland

General Dental Council (GDC) (1997) *The First Five Years: The Undergraduate Dental Curriculum*

Gleeson, F (1997) *Assessment of the objective structured long examination record (OSLER)*, AMEE Guide No 9, Dundee, Scotland

General Medical Council (GMC) (1993) *Tomorrow's Doctors: Recommendations on Undergraduate Medical Education* [Online] http://www.gmc-uk.org/meded/meded-frameset.htm

GMC (2000) *Revalidation* [Online] http://www.gmc-uk.org/revalidation/index.html

Grounlund, N E and Linn, R L (1985) *Measurement and Evaluation of Teaching*, 6th edn, Collier Macmillan Publishers, New York

Hammond, E J *et al* (1998) Multiple-choice examinations: adopting an evidence-based approach to exam technique, *Anaesthesia*, **53**, pp 1105–08

Harden, R M (1979) How to assess students: an overview, *Medical Teacher*, **1** (2), pp 65–70

Harden, R M and Gleeson, F A (1979) Assessment of Clinical Competence Using Objective Structured Clinical Examination, *Medical Education*, **13**, pp 39–54

Harden, R M and Crosby, J R (2001) *The good teacher is more than a lecturer – the twelve roles of the teacher*, AMEE Guide No 20, *Medical Teacher*, **22**, pp 334–47

Harding Rains, A J (1996) *1001 Multiple Choice Questions and Answers in Surgery*, 4th edn, Chapman and Hall, London

Khan, K S, Davies, D A and Gupta, J K (2001) Formative self-assessment using multiple true-false questions on the Internet: feedback according to confidence about correct knowledge, *Medical Teacher*, **23** (2), pp 158–63

King, W, Gray, P F and Hossacks, J D (1992) Peer marking of technical reports, *CAP-ability*, **2**, pp 20–25

Mahalski, P A (1992) Essay writing: do study manuals give relevant advice?, *Higher Education*, **24** (1), pp 113–32

Mavis, B E, Cole, B L and Hoppe, R B (2001) A survey of student assessment in US medical schools: the balance of breadth versus fidelity, *Teaching and Learning in Medicine*, **13** (2), pp 74–79

Mossey, P A and Newton, J P (2001) The structured clinical operative test (SCOT) in dental competency assessment, *British Dental Journal*, **190** (7), pp 387–90

Newble, D I and Jaeger, K (1983) The effect of assessment and examination on the learning of medical students, *Medical Education*, **17**, pp 165–67

Odgen, G R, Green, M and Ker, J S (2000) The use of interprofessional peer examiners in objective structured clinical examinations: can dental students act as examiners?, *British Dental Journal*, **189** (3), pp 160–64

Premadasa, I G (1993) A reappraisal of the use of multiple choice questions, *Medical Teacher*, **15** (2–3), pp 237–42

Rennie, S C and Crosby, J R (2002) Really Good Stuff – The SCOT in Medicine, *Medical Education*, in press

Rolfe, I and McPherson, J (1995) Formative Assessment: how am I doing?, *Lancet*, **345**, pp 837–39

Rowntree, D (1987) *Assessing Students: How shall we know them?*, Kogan Page, London

Scrivens, M (1967) The methodology of evaluation, in *Perspectives of curriculum evaluation*, ed R W Tyler *et al*, Rand McNally, Chicago

Smith, R M (1993) The triple jump examination as an assessment tool in the problem based medical curriculum at the University of Hawaii, *Academic Medicine*, **68** (5), pp 366–72

Snadden, D, Thomas, M and Challis, M (1999) *Portfolio-based learning and assessment*, AMEE Education Guide No 11 (revised), Dundee, Scotland

Torrance, H (1995) *Evaluating authentic assessment: Problems and possibilities in new approaches to assessment*, OUP, Buckingham

van der Vleuten, C P, Verwijnen, G M and Wijnen, W H (1996) Fifteen years of experience with progress testing in a problem based learning curriculum, *Medical Teacher*, **18** (2), pp 103–10

Recommended reading

Validity

Grounlund, N E and Linn, R L (1985a) *Measurement and Evaluation of Teaching*, 6th edn, Collier Macmillan Publishers, New York, Chapter 3, pp 47–76

Reliability

Grounlund, N E and Linn, R L (1985b) *Measurement and Evaluation of Teaching*, 6th edn, Collier Macmillan Publishers, New York, Chapter 4, pp 77–108

OSLER

Gleeson, F (1997) *Assessment of the objective structured long examination record (OSLER)*, AMEE Guide No 9, Dundee, Scotland

Portfolio assessment

Snadden, D, Thomas, M and Challis, M (1999) *Portfolio-based learning and assessment*, AMEE Education Guide No 11 (revised), Dundee, Scotland

6

Large group teaching and interactive lectures

Iain Robbé

Preamble

In our MDV undergraduate education we have all often attended lectures and our postgraduate work also offers many opportunities to attend lectures and to deliver them. In this chapter I shall discuss how to make lectures more effective, whether you are attending or you are facilitating them. As a working definition, I will consider a large group that is identified arbitrarily as more than 30 people and the median time of the lecture is 60 minutes, although it could be as short as 30 minutes. I shall use the word 'audience' for the adult learners at the lecture – you might be a lecturer facilitating the lecture or an adult learner in the audience.

Exercise 1

Before you read further into this chapter, please think of the lectures you have attended or facilitated in the past year and identify four positive issues and four negative issues. These issues might relate to the lecturer, the audience, the content or the resources.

Positive issues:
(1)
(2)
(3)
(4)

Negative issues:
(1)
(2)
(3)
(4)

The education literature (Bligh, 2000; Newble and Cannon, 1994) suggests that amongst the issues you will have identified are factors related to the:

- **lecturer** – positive issues: enthusiastic, arrives on time, varies tone of speech, pauses and highlights, moves around, responds to the audience, confident;
  negative issues: speaks quietly, reads from a script, avoids eye contact with the audience, hurries speech towards the end, leaves swiftly;
- **audience** – positive issues: involved by being spoken to, interested in the content, willing to talk in the break up periods;
  negative issues: microsleeps affect everyone, attention span falls with time, arriving late, talking to each other across the facilitator;
- **content** – positive issues: principles linked to new information or reinforcing older information, well-prepared examples and humour, clear structure;
  negative issues: too complex or too simplistic, repetition of readily available information;
- **resources** – positive issues: use of a range of methods to break up the lecture, handouts (might be comprehensive, outline, or key points), slides or overheads (not both);
  negative issues: illegible audio-visual aids, flip chart is too small for a lecture.

I shall return to these issues later in the chapter but they will serve as reminders of your experiences of recent lectures while you are reading this chapter.

Introduction

Lectures to promote active learning

The objectives of this chapter are:

- to build on your experiences of lectures so that in future you will make lectures more effective;
- to use a taxonomy based on Gagné's work (Curzon, 1990) so that you can promote active learning in lectures;
- to structure the chapter as if it was being presented as a lecture involving not only the lecturer but also the audience, content issues, and resources where possible.

Effectiveness in lectures

Generally, the literature has achieved a consensus that lectures are an appropriate teaching method for delivering information (Bligh, 2000; Newble and Cannon, 1994), particularly when the contents need to be synthesized, eg, in screening for prostate cancer, linking the physiology of cancer growth with the anatomy of the prostate, and the ethics of diagnosing a symptomless disease that has unproven treatment regimens. Lectures are appropriate for developing an interest in a subject particularly from a special perspective, eg, the public health benefits of stopping smoking contrasted with the pleasures from smoking for a stressed, unemployed single mother. Lectures are also useful for short-term memorization, eg, revision lectures before examinations (Curzon, 1990).

Lectures are less appropriate for promoting thinking about the use of knowledge (Coles, 1998), for altering attitudes, values or behaviour (Bligh, 2000) and for long-term memorization (Curzon, 1990).

Planning a lecture with active learning

The exercise in the preamble was included in this chapter for two reasons. Firstly, it is useful in a lecture to gain the audience's attention as soon as possible and asking you to do something should have gained your attention. Secondly, it is important to stimulate your recall of previous experiences and you will have immediately identified various contexts for positive and negative issues in lectures (David *et al*, 1998). You are likely to relate many aspects of learning in lectures in the rest of this chapter to these contexts.

A widely used taxonomy in educational design is Gagné's 'Nine Events of Instruction' (Curzon, 1990), which, in my experience is more andragogical than the word 'instruction' would suggest and the events are useful in lecture planning. Also Gagné's events draw on cognitive education psychology (Curzon, 1990) with the emphasis on the learners and their contexts, their mental processing of information, and their uses of knowledge to make decisions and to be effective. The nine events are:

1. gaining attention;
2. informing learners of objectives;
3. stimulating recall;
4. presenting stimulus material;
5. providing learner guidance;
6. eliciting performance;
7. providing feedback;
8. assessing performance;
9. enhancing retention and transfer to your own contexts.

This chapter is structured as if it was being delivered as a lecture, ie:

- **Preamble** – seeks to gain your attention and to stimulate your recall of relevant experiences.
- **Introduction: Lectures to promote active learning** – informs you of the objectives. If I was facilitating a series of lectures then I would remind the audience of previous lectures, partly to stimulate recall and also to link the content to the audience's needs. An advance organizer can be provided for the audience before the lecture (Bligh, 2000) to prepare the way for the content of the lecture, typically by reminding the learners of known concepts and linking to the material in the lecture. In my experience, medical undergraduates rarely read and reflect on the organizer before the lecture, often due to the pressures on their time and the number of lectures they have to attend. Postgraduates are more likely to think about the contents of an advance organizer but they too find it difficult to give time to it before a single lecture – they are more likely to reflect if the organizer is to be part of a session or sessions ie, two hours or longer.

  The objectives can also be labelled 'draft' as the audience might be able to express particular needs. For example, I gave out a questionnaire at the end of the first lecture on health promotion to 150 medical students. Thirty per cent responded by completing the questionnaire immediately and amongst other issues they chose topics for the second lecture so I started the second lecture by showing them their 'votes' for specific health promotion issues and using those issues as examples in the content. The draft objectives became more specific to their interests, eg, contact tracing in sexually transmitted diseases, healthy foods for low-income families, chemoprophylaxis in meningococcal disease.
- **Effectiveness in lectures** – the above section entitled 'Effectiveness in lectures' was written to provide you with stimulus material about the best uses for lectures.
- **Planning a lecture with active learning** – provides further stimulus material and learning guidance within a framework. The education literature (Bligh, 2000; Newble and Cannon, 1994) is consistent with the view that learning is enhanced when the learners can interact with each other and with the facilitator, ie, when there is active learning. There are many ways to promote active learning in lectures and the challenge is twofold. Firstly the facilitator wishes to provide opportunities for active learning in the large group and secondly the learning should be deep and not surface learning.

  For the purposes of promoting deep learning in lectures, Biggs's work (1993) is particularly relevant as he argues that surface and deep learning depend on the context, the task, and the information processing by the individuals. Surface learning occurs when new knowledge adds to existing understood knowledge without further understanding. In contrast, deep learning seeks to integrate new knowledge into existing knowledge, to maximize understanding, and to modify knowledge. The differences are illustrated in the following example in Table 6.1.

Table 6.1 The differences between deep and surface learning

lecture: facilitator has the same task of delivering information to medical students; indicates two different contexts			
Task	**Context**	**Information Processing**	**Learning**
facilitator delivers information about the routes of the three main branches of the trigeminal nerve	common viva topic when the student is asked 'describe the routes of the...'	rote learning with the viva in mind to avoid humiliation and failure	surface
facilitator delivers information about the routes of the three main branches of the trigeminal nerve	facial trauma is a common presentation in the casualty department	relates the routes to the trauma, thinks how to test for sensory and motor damage, thinks how surgeon will plan treatment	deep
lecture: facilitator has the task of discussing a subject from a special perspective with medical students; gives more mention of ethics in one lecture; indicates same contexts to students			
facilitator considers effects from smoking at the three levels of the individual, local society, population in general; brief mention of ethics lectures	general practitioner advising pregnant, stressed, single mother	rote learning about the three levels in order to explain them to the patient, or in an essay exam. Notes ethical issues without new understanding. fear of failure is strong	surface
facilitator considers effects from smoking at the three levels of the individual, local society, population in general; recalls ethics lectures and relates them to public health	general practitioner advising pregnant, stressed, single mother	relates the three levels to ethics -- patient autonomy, beneficence, and population benefits; modifies existing knowledge to offer alternatives to the patient; accepts uncertainty of patient choice	deep

The many dimensions to adult learning are beyond the objectives of this chapter but there are relevant sources of further information including the learning styles and internal information processing linked to an individual's psychology (Jonassen and Grabowski, 1993), learning approaches (Marton and Säljö, 1997; Newble and Entwistle, 1986), and Biggs's work (1993) on learning processes.

Further headings in this chapter will include, amongst others: **Exercise 2** – eliciting performance; **Delivery of content** – providing feedback and assessing performance; **Variations in teaching methods** and **Conclusion** – enhancing retention and transferring to your own contexts.

Exercise 2

Please think of the following scenario – you have agreed to facilitate a lecture for 40 postgraduates for one hour and you have defined a set of four to five objectives. Now you are wrestling with decisions about the methods to teach the content. Please brainstorm to think of a few advantages and disadvantages of these methods:

Method (Brown and Atkins, 1988)	**Advantages**	**Disadvantages**
traditional: wide reading of possible topic areas, identify linked topics, key stages, create a logical structure eg, health promotion in cardio-vascular diseases with primary, secondary and tertiary prevention		
problem-based: use a clinical patient with multiple system involvement eg, diabetes mellitus		
sequencing: take a scientific approach ie, several case studies lead to an inductive hypothesis that is tested eg, cluster of cases of new variant Creutzfeldt-Jakob diseases, hypothesis of an infectious agent, tracked down and identified the prion from bovine spongiform encephalopathy (BSE)		

Delivery of content

The purposes of Exercise 2 were to break up the reading of this chapter so that you could be more active and to draw on your experiences of lecture methods, ie, eliciting a performance from you and offering feedback from me. Firstly you will have noted the information about the context, ie, your audience will be 40 people and they are postgraduates. Also you have agreed four to five objectives, which is about the maximum you can address in one lecture of an hour.

Turning to my feedback on your thoughts on advantages and disadvantages of the methods for teaching the content – the traditional method is logical and well-structured but it might not engage the audience, particularly if they do not have relevant experiences. The problem-centred method, particularly if it is linked to cases seen by the audience, will often encourage active learning and it promotes alternative solutions that can be discussed, drawing on the audience's experiences. The sequencing method can also engage the audience, particularly if there is a topical issue such as BSE or meningitis amongst university students and there is a chain of reasoning that leads to conclusions.

The structuring of the lecture can be based on Gagné's events and they are linked to the experiential learning cycle that is becoming increasingly relevant to our continued professional development in our medical, dental or veterinary vocations. The experiential learning cycle has its origins in Kolb's work (1984) outlined in Chapter 4 (see Figure 4.4)

Stages in the learning cycle

This chapter started by asking you to think of your experiences in lectures; to outline your concrete experience, which is at Stage 1 in the cycle. During the subsequent reading you have been entering in to Stage 2 with reflections on your experiences. Those reflections have possibly been linked to theories and concepts of adult learning, particularly deep and active learning, and if you make generalizations about these links then you will be moving to Stage 3, theorizing with abstract concepts and generalizations about the experience. Finally, you might test the generalizations and new ideas for the practice of lectures in your work – Stage 4.

Breaking up the monologue

The next issue in the facilitation of the lecture concerns the use of resources. There are many education texts that give advice about audio-visual aids, particularly Heinich *et al* (1996), Newble and Cannon (1994), and Reigluth (1983). However, I wish to concentrate on ways of breaking up the monologue tendency in a lecture so that deep learning is facilitated. In addition to promoting deep learning, breaking up the monologue is also useful for providing feedback, combating the microsleeps that everyone in the audience experiences, and for reducing attention decline. It has been well-identified that attention declines steadily after the first 5–10 minutes of a 60-minute lecture to reach a minimum at about 20 minutes before increasing steadily to nearly the starting level in the last five minutes (Bligh,

2000; Giles *et al*, 1982). However, as Bligh has discussed, variations in the teaching methods can markedly increase the attention levels as well as preventing microsleeps from reducing learning.

Variations in teaching methods

Buzz groups

Groups of two to six members discuss a clear task set by the facilitator within the lecture for a few minutes. For example, identify the three main causes of breast cancer in women. These groups are useful when too many people wish to contribute or some are too reticent to participate in front of 30 or more people. Undergraduates generally do not like talking in the plenary even when reporting back from a buzz group so I tend to offer the answers after they have discussed the task, eg, 'I anticipate that you will have identified these causes a, b, and c. Many people think x is a cause but there is little evidence.' Postgraduates are more comfortable giving feedback and for them buzz groups are particularly useful for obtaining the views of quieter learners.

Mechanical response systems

These systems require software and individual handsets for each person and the lecturer can pose planned questions and the learners can respond (Roy, 1996). They can answer with true, false, don't know answers or they can choose from several items from a list.These systems are useful for giving immediate feedback to the learners about their responses and the lecturer who might be able to reply immediately, eg, when the difference between incidence and prevalence was not understood after an explanation, then I was able to rephrase the definition before proceeding further with the lecture.

The systems can also be useful to follow changes over time. For example, a cohort of oncologists showed an increased use of evidence-based literature between two meetings six months apart. Generally these systems have been well received as they encourage deep thinking and particularly they enable links to be made between concepts and new information (Roy, 1996). Thus, in the above example about the trigeminal cranial nerve, deep learning could be inferred if there were correct responses to questions that required application of the facts about the routes of the nerve and the effects of trauma on sensation from different parts of the face as the nerve carries facial sensations, and on mastication functions as the nerve controls motor functions to the muscles of mastication. The systems take longer to use than direct questions and a technician is usually needed to resolve problems, particularly if the lecturer wishes to pose unplanned questions.

Pauses

Silences are generally discomforting in our society but they can be helpful in lectures to allow time for note-taking or for the individuals to think alone while they review their notes or summarize (Coles, 1998). They also give me an opportunity to look round the room to check for nods of understanding, puzzled expressions or loss of attention. I can show the audience that I am trying to think of them. Occasionally a subgroup can be 'lost' from the lecture and start talking amongst themselves. Once this situation begins to distract others in the audience, a pause can embarrass the talkers into listening quietly or participating in the break-up methods. It damages the constructive atmosphere if I have to ask for silence but reluctantly I sometimes do ask the talkers to be quiet out of consideration for those people who want to listen.

Questions and discussions

The lecturer can try and encourage learners to ask questions at any time. Generally, undergraduates do not interrupt and even postgraduates tend not to intervene, and when they do, the question can derail the train of thought of the lecturer and others in the audience. I have found that the use of quiz questions that are integral to the content has helped people to think for themselves and to even talk to their neighbours when asked a specific question during the lecture. These questions help to link issues, eg, a question about an opaque mass on a chest x-ray: is it a cancer, tuberculosis, or a foreign body? I can then link the anatomy of the lung to the pathology of lung cancer to cigarettes and primary prevention. These questions also enable me to identify issues for other lectures to the same audience or in subsequent years.

Conclusion

Exercise 3

In order to provide you with some further feedback and possibly to assess your performance in lectures, please could you think of any experiences in lectures in your career that were particularly effective in stimulating deep learning ? Why do you remember these experiences – a charismatic lecturer, clever use of resources such as a stoical patient or a mechanical response system, a particularly enthusiastic audience, a subject that is dear to your heart? Could you do something to emulate these memorable experiences in future lectures?

Summaries usually occur at the end of the lecture although they can be useful to reinforce the completion of an objective during the lecture, eg, '… there are three specific issues that we have discussed about primary prevention; the issues are then reiterated… ; now we shall move on to secondary prevention'.

Typically though, the summary brings the lecture to a definite conclusion by reinforcing the objectives and how they have been achieved. The summary also tries to end the lecture in a positive way. In this chapter the objectives were:

- To build on your experiences of lectures so that in future you will make lectures more effective. I hope that reading this text and participating in the exercises has given you contexts for your lecture planning and facilitation in the future.
- To use a taxonomy based on Gagné's work (Curzon, 1990) so that you can promote active learning in lectures. I trust the issue of active learning had high validity for you and that you might use the taxonomy or modify it for your lectures. This point links to Gagné's events concerning the enhancement of learning retention and the transfer to your own contexts.
- To structure the chapter as if it was being presented as a lecture. Your views on the effectiveness of this structure will be of interest to the editors and of even more interest to me. I hope you will provide me with feedback via the contributor's address at the front of this book.

Exercise 4

Please think of this chapter as if it had been a lecture and assess it in terms of how close items in each of the four areas were to the 'target' or centre ie, the closer to the centre indicates an item was used more effectively or favourably than if you place it on the periphery.

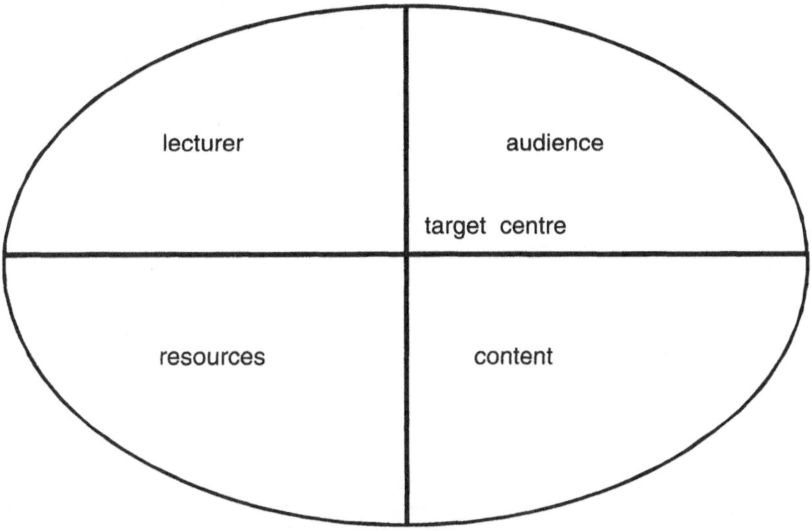

Figure 6.1 Lecture emphasis

References

Biggs, J B (1993) What do Inventories of Students' Learning Processes really Measure? A theoretical review and clarification, *British J Educational Psychology*, **63**, pp 3–19.

Bligh, D A (2000) *What's the Use of Lectures ?*, 1st edn USA, Jossey-Bass, San Francisco

Brown, G and Atkins, M (1988) *Effective Teaching in Higher Education*, Routledge, London

Coles, C R (1998) How Students Learn: the Process of Learning, in *Medical Education in the Millennium*, eds B Jolly and L Rees, Oxford Medical, Oxford

Curzon, L B (1990) *Teaching in Further Education*, 4th edn, Cassell Education, London

David, T J *et al* (1998) Problem based Learning as an Alternative to Lecture based Continuing Medical Education, *Journal Royal Society Medicine*, **91**, pp 626–30

Giles, R M *et al* (1982) Recall of Lecture Information: a Question of What, When and Where, *Medical Education*, **16**, pp 264–68

Heinich, R *et al* (1996) *Instructional Media and Technologies for Learning*, 5th edn, Prentice Hall, Englewood Cliffs, New Jersey

Jonassen, D H and Grabowski, B L (1993) *Handbook of Individual Differences, Learning, and Instruction*, Lawrence Erlbaum, London

Kolb, D A (1984) *Experiential Learning. Experience as the Source of Learning and Development*, Prentice-Hall, Englewood Cliffs, New Jersey

Marton, F and Säljö, R (1997) Approaches to Learning, in *The Experience of Learning*, eds F Marton, D Hounsell and N J Entwistle, 2nd edn, Scottish Academic Press, Edinburgh

Newble, D I and Entwistle, N J (1986). Learning Styles and Approaches: Implications for Medical Education, *Medical Education*, **20**, pp 162–75

Newble, D I and Cannon, R (1994) *A Handbook for Medical Teachers*, 3rd edn, Kluwer Academic, London

Reigluth, C (1983) *Instructional Design, Theories and Models*, Lawrence Erlbaum, Hillsdale, New Jersey

Roy, K H (1996) Pilot Investigation of the Utility of a Student Response System in Medical Student Lectures, *J Audiovisual Media in Medicine*, **19** (1), pp 27–32

7

Learning in small groups and problem-based learning

Joy Crosby

Introduction

The advantages of small group learning

Small group learning is often the most meaningful learning experienced by students and should be utilized in all curricula. It should be characterized by the active participation of all members of the group, involvement of the group towards a communal task (Tiberius, 1999) and time for the group to reflect on its learning (Kolb, 1984). These logistics limit the number of students that can work in a small group, so that its size will depend on the skill of the facilitator and also the group dynamics. The six main advantages of small group learning are explained below:

- **It enhances a deep approach to learning**
  Biggs (1999) describes a continuum of learning activities that students can undertake from low-level memorizing, note-taking and recognizing, to increasingly higher levels, which include relating, applying, generation of ideas, theorizing and reflecting. All these types of learning are relevant for all students at different times, but students studying for the professions will need to be continually using the higher learning activities of applying theory to practice and planning complex treatment options to become successful practitioners.
  Biggs (1999) states that passive teaching, like the delivery of lectures, will tend to encourage the lower-order memorizing and note-taking. Active teaching, on the other hand, through small group enquiry methods stimulates the higher-

order activities and demands that students engage in these (Entwistle, Thompson and Tait, 1992). Good teaching therefore entails ensuring that students use their higher-level cognitive processes. When students use simple memorizing, recording and note-taking instead of the higher-order processes they are using a surface approach to learning (Biggs, 1999). If students are using this learning approach with a piece of text, they will tend to concentrate anxiously on the facts and details that might be asked, to get it over with quickly. They tend to remember a list of disjointed facts and often do not get the point the author is trying to convey. An alternative is the deep approach, where students burrow beneath the surface of the text to interpret its meaning. They will see the overall picture and be able to assemble enough detail to make out the point the author is trying to make. Curricula should attempt to move from the encouragement of rote learning to a deeper approach to learning. Small group learning may better achieve this aim than more solitary methods of learning.

- **It develops generic skills**
  Within MDV medicine there is an expectation that a graduate will have certain generic and transferable skills. One of the major skills required of all clinical practitioners is the ability to communicate. In small groups students have to communicate to learn. The student can develop even the basic rudiments of communication skills through discussion with peers. Small groups give students the opportunity to listen to others and also to express themselves (Walton, 1997). In addition, the ability to present a coherent argument, defend a position and give feedback to others can be developed (Entwistle, Thompson and Tait, 1992). The ability to reflect on their own individual input as well as that of other group members is an important attribute of professionalism (see Chapter 12).

  When students have graduated they will invariably have to work as a member of a team and work collaboratively with colleagues in order to ensure the best possible care for patients or clients. They will have to be able to cope with individuals they may not like or respect, who would dominate or not contribute. In using small groups a student may be better prepared to function effectively as a member of a team.
- **It encourages students to take responsibility for learning**
  In medical education, in the early 1980s, a movement from teacher-centred to more student-centred modes of learning encouraged students to take greater responsibility and autonomy for their own learning (Harden, Sowden and Dunn, 1984). This can be facilitated through small group work.
- **It promotes adult learning styles**
  Small group work mirrors advanced learning situations that are more likely to occur in the postgraduate setting. Certainly, departmental/ward/unit meetings tend to adopt a small group approach rather than that of a formal lecture. Students may benefit from small group work in order to equip themselves with skills to function appropriately in this type of setting.

- **It allows individuals to work in different ways**
  Individuals have different learning styles, which can be identified by questionnaire to produce a learning style inventory (Honey and Mumford, 1982). Some students will find the lecture an advantageous way to learn whilst others may prefer reading books and journals, computer-assisted learning (CAL) or talking informally with friends. Diversity of teaching methods can be encouraged to satisfy more preferences, but most effective learners are those who can operate in a wide range of styles (Renzulli and Smith *et al*, 2002). So students should be encouraged to consolidate their strengths and work on weaknesses to change their learning behaviour.
- **It stimulates student motivation**
  Working in small groups has been found to increase short-term motivation and satisfaction with learning (Brookfield, 1988). Motivation is one of the key elements necessary for meaningful learning and active involvement motivates individuals to learn (Tiberius, 1999). It has also been found that students involved in small group work have more favourable attitudes and greater persistence to learning (Springer, Stanne and Donovan, 1999).

Factors to consider when running small groups

Careful consideration should be given before embarking on a small group programme. Small group work is not an easy option for members of staff or students as it must be a focussed activity with clear learning outcomes. The small group activity should be an integral part of the overall curriculum. Staff need to be skilled at both writing the stimulus material and the facilitation of the small groups. The environment must be conducive to small group work and in order to promote interaction the group should be positioned in a circle or U shape, possibly formed around a table. The room should be comfortable, without distractions, but with the required resources; for example, written literature, flip chart and pens. If a lecture theatre is the only space available, then alternative lecture-based strategies for active learning should be considered (see Chapter 6).

Group composition

Once a decision has been made to utilize small group work the composition of the group must be considered. Generally, in undergraduate education, a good mix of students of different gender, ethnic origin, ability and possibly age, offers the potential for a greater range of perspectives and variety in experiences of learning. One issue for concern is how frequently a small group should be changed during the duration of a course. Becoming used to forming and reforming small groups may be a beneficial learning experience but this must be weighed against cases where groups are functioning well and students are learning from each other so learning will be disrupted if the group is disbanded.

Setting ground rules

When a small group meets for the first time it must set ground rules. If the members of the group do not know each other 'ice-breakers' can be used too allow the members to get used to each other and start to work together. All groups should recognize and set ground rules for the functioning of the group. These should be made explicit at the start of the formation of the group, but may be renegotiated as the group develops. The ground rules should be considered as a group and not just imposed by the tutor. Rules may include:

- that everyone should attend;
- that everyone should participate;
- that no contribution should be ridiculed;
- that all sensitive information should be kept confidential;
- that individuals will not be interrupted when talking;
- that everyone will do any preparatory work and present material when required.

Assessment and evaluating small groups

Before embarking on a programme of small group work consideration should be given to assessment and evaluation. If the focus of small group work is knowledge then traditional paper-based assessment may be appropriate. For team-working skills peer assessment may be advantageous. Peers can identify whether they feel comfortable working with a student and if they are able to communicate effectively with other members of the group (see Chapter 5).

Evaluation of both the student and staff experience can be invaluable in the development of a programme of learning. Students may be asked to rate the session and the facilitator:

- Did you know the purpose of the session?
- Were you able to ask questions?
- Did you have an opportunity to contribute to the session?
- Did everyone participate?
- Did you feel you had responsibility for your learning?

In addition, there should be focus on the perceived quality of learning. Evidence should be collected to illuminate aspects that may improve learning by asking:

- What aspects of the experience seemed to promote learning?
- What aspects of the experience seemed to limit learning?
- What aspects could be modified to improve the quality of learning?

If this is a new experience for staff, their attitudes and opinions of the session may also be sought. It may also be advantageous to peer review sessions for inexperienced staff, in order to identify strengths and weaknesses, to inform future practice.

Types of small group work

There are a whole variety of small group methods that may be used singly or together to facilitate learning. The resources available will largely determine the choice of technique.

Tutorial

This is perhaps one of the most widely used methods of small group work. The primary use of the tutorial is to develop an understanding of a topic. Tutorials should also promote debating and interpersonal skills. In the tutorial a teacher is responsible for setting stimulus questions, which students must consider prior to the tutorial session. Students should come to the session with prepared answers. The questions may be very specific or more open. For example, a closed question may be 'List the different approaches to pain management'. A more open question may include a case scenario where the students are asked to consider a differential diagnosis, investigations and management. During the sessions students should be encouraged to answer the questions and discuss them with their peers. A well-run and structured tutorial may result in the facilitator saying little. The main role of the facilitator should be to pose questions and to guide the discussion. At the end of the session students should identify if there are areas that they still need to consider.

Seminar

The seminar aims to develop student understanding of a topic and research ability. The student should make a presentation in a coherent manner and critically discuss a topic. The remit is generally broader than for tutorial questions. For example, 'Consider and present a strategy for managing an outbreak of an infectious disease'. Raaheim (1991) suggests that presenting material is one of the most effective ways to learn. All students should prepare for the general discussion, which should take 50 per cent of the available time.

Free discussion and brain storming

The free discussion group involves no formal presentation and is often used to discuss affective and contentious topics, for example, 'Should private practice be encouraged?'. It allows the group to discuss all possible avenues and so permits appreciation of other people's views.

Brainstorming is a small group method adopted primarily for the generation of ideas. Participants may be posed with a question for which several options may be viable. For example, 'How could cancerous cells be removed from the body?' The group should suggest possible solutions; for example, cut it out, dissolve them with chemicals, irradiate them, etc. At this point no discussion of the value of the solution should be made. Once all solutions have been generated the group should discuss each solution and group those they feel are of value. In this way themes are generated. In a further small group session the value of the solutions may be explored.

Role play

Role play is useful in exploring and developing strategies to deal with difficult emotional situations. A role playing exercise may be conducted in two ways. Firstly, a student may be requested to enact a situation that they may be exposed to in their future practice; for example, how to break bad news to someone. The student will be briefed regarding the scenario. For example, 'You have just received results indicating that the patient has irreparable damage to the spinal cord resulting in paraplegia – inform the patient/client of the findings'. In order for the situation to be realistic the student has to impart the information to an individual who is able to act in an appropriate manner. Sometimes a simulated patient, either trained actors, or other group member may be given a script outlining the scenario and the behaviour they wish to express, for example, shock, anger, etc. This type of approach allows the student to practice a difficult skill in a protected environment before being expected to demonstrate this ability in a real situation.

The second approach is the enactment of how a patient or relative may feel in a given situation. The intention of this approach is to allow the students some insight into how an individual may feel. This awareness may help them deal more sensitively with a patient in that situation in the future. It is important that at the end of the session, students stop playing the role they have been assigned and return to 'being a student'. Some students may take the role seriously and may feel anger after playing the 'angry patient'. A debriefing session following role play can allow the student presenting work or playing in a role play to identify positive aspects of the work or interaction. A small group observing role play can offer to identify any further points missed and finally the facilitator should input positive points noted. The student should then highlight areas for improvement, followed by the rest of the group and finally the tutor, if necessary. This process is beneficial as it focusses initially on good aspects that are frequently overlooked and secondly gives the student and the rest of the group responsibility for evaluating performance.

Clinical skills

The majority of clinical teaching is often conducted in small groups. Whilst the location of the teaching (wards, clinics, clinical skills centres and ambulatory teaching areas) and the authenticity of the patient (real patient, simulated patient or model) may vary, the principles of the small group work are the same. The small group instructional skills of clinical teachers are considered one of the most important determinants of effective clinical teaching (Mcleod and Harden, 1985). Six key steps may be considered as shown in Table 7.1.

Table 7.1 Six steps in demonstration of a practical skill

Activity	**Example**
tutor explains the skill	outline of procedure
tutor demonstrates skills	inserting a venflon (using a student, patient or model)
tutor demonstrates and describes actions	explanation of what is happening
student attempts the skill	inserts a venflon
teacher/group give constructive feedback	good points and points for improvement
students practice (repetition and feedback)	inserts a venflon

With clinical small group work it is imperative that all students can observe the demonstration. Competence in a skill will not be acquired immediately. Practice and repetition are required to acquire competence (Cox and Ewan, 1988).

Which small group technique to use?

The types of group work adopted depend on the outcomes expected from learning. Table 7.2 below summarizes some outcomes, the possible type of group to use, resources required and some key issues to consider.

Table 7.2 Small group types

Outcomes Expected	Type of Group	Resources Required	Key Issues
increase in deep understanding	tutorial seminar problem-based learning	stimulus material, eg patient cases resources for researching the topic	ensuring students prepared for the sessions ensuring that the small group session allows student expression of learning
awareness and appreciations of attitudinal issues	role play free discussion group	stimulus material, eg scripts, required to ensure adequate and realistic briefing of students	emotions may be heightened and disagreement may ensue – some individuals may be reticent about contributing
development of team working skills	most methods that emphasize group collaboration seminar work problem-based learning	clear group task method of identifying individual contribution	awareness of group dynamics and clarity regarding the roles expected
enhanced creativity and problem-solving skills	problem-based learning brain storming	clear statement of problem flip chart or white board resource material	a supporting and trusting environment is required
development of clinical skills communication and consultation skills	demonstration and practice role playing	patients (real or simulated) or models	consider the implications of using real or simulated patients

The facilitator

Facilitation means 'the work involved in ensuring that the right structures and processes exist for helping the group to meet its agreed objectives and in helping the group members to identify and overcome problems communicating with one another in managing emotion' (Elwyn, Greenhalgh and MacFarlen, 2001). The term facilitator therefore provides a more accurate description than teacher or tutor for the appropriate leadership of a small group. Facilitators, without training, tend to adopt one of three styles:

- In the **autonomous style** the facilitator may allow the group to make its own decisions, right or wrong. This may eventually be the ideal learning situation but is also fraught with difficulties especially with young groups who have not yet formed as a functioning effective unit. The facilitator must be confident in the abilities of the group.
- The **autocratic style** is the least preferred, where the facilitator makes all the key decisions. This may be useful when a group is just forming or if the group needs to be reformed. This style of facilitation is not encouraged as it takes away the students' responsibility for their learning.
- The **democratic style** of facilitation attempts to give each member of the group, including the facilitator, an equal say in how the group functions.

Irrespective of the natural style of facilitation an individual can be taught to facilitate a group. The facilitator has two main functions: to ensure that the task is achieved and to ensure the group cohesion is maintained in order to fulfil the task (Jacques, 1996).

Task functions

To ensure that the group completes the task the facilitator must be aware of the nature of the small group work and its place in the overall programme – the facilitator has to appreciate why the group is meeting in the wider context of the curriculum. The overall MDV course coordinator must share the wider picture indicating the need for the small group sessions. If this key step is not taken small group work may be unsuccessfully implemented.

The facilitator must also be aware of the availability of stimulus material – frequently students need stimulus material to consider. The material should be well thought out and produced in an accessible, timely manner. For example, a clinical case scenario described must be free of errors. A management strategy, for instance, must be set at a level appropriate to the student's learning.

The facilitator should outline the task, the time and the resources available to the students. The duration of the session may be outside the control of the facilitator but timing is crucial to task completion.

Active roles of the facilitator

During the session the facilitator has many roles, which include:

- Questioning the students' understanding. Questioning and the answering of questions is a key aspect of small group learning. The facilitator should not only ask questions, but also encourage students to ask questions regarding the tasks in hand.

- Clarifying issues. Where necessary the facilitator should clarify areas of misunderstanding and confusion.
- Summarizing achievements. At the end of the session the attainment by the group should be summarized.

Maintaining the cohesion of a group

Perhaps the most challenging role of the facilitator is to maintain the cohesion of the group. In order to fulfil this task the facilitator should be aware of the different phases a group may experience. Groups go through different stages of development. Thelen and Dickerman (1949) were the first to attempt to describe group development. In the 1960s, Bion described groups as being in one of three stages, stage 1: flight, stage 2: fight and stage 3: unite (Bion, 1961). These equate in part to, perhaps the most widely used, descriptors of group development devised by Tuckman. Tuckman and Jensen (1977) proposed five different phases: forming, norming, storming, performing and disbanding, as shown in Table 7.3.

Table 7.3 Group development

Forming	Polite stage, where group members are getting to know each other and are on their best behaviour. An icebreaker could be used to speed up movement through this stage.
Norming	Ground rules are set, formal or informal, in order to function effectively. Introducing formal ground rules is advantageous and is likely to reduce the impact of the storming phase.
Forming and storming are encapsulated in Bion's flight stage where the participants may rather be elsewhere.	
Storming	The group members disagree with each other about how they should achieve the task and how they should behave. Open conflict, arguments, may ensue. Storming may not been seen openly but members of the group may be unhappy (Bion's fight stage).
Performing	The effectively functioning group where all members are involved and fulfilling the task (Bion's unite stage).
Disbanding	The process of the group breaking up. This may be tinged with sadness.

It is useful to understand the dynamics of a group in order to place the experience in some context. During the storming phase, the request to move students to a different group should be resisted. This request may come from a student or from other members of the group. Most requests are related to personal differences within the group. The request should be resisted for three reasons. Firstly, MDV professionals seldom have the luxury in working life to alter the groups they work in. Working through interpersonal problems is an important skill to develop. Secondly, the problems originally stated may be replicated in the new group. Thirdly, a new group member may disrupt an already performing group. However, there are no absolutes so whereas personal differences may not be an adequate reason, bullying and victimization should be taken seriously.

To maintain the cohesion of a group the facilitator should be good at observing, be a diplomat, challenge students and be prepared to address difficult situations. Observing what is happening in a group is paramount. Even the smallest things are important, and relate to the learner as an individual:

- Where are people sitting? Has anyone deliberately taken a dominant or reclusive chair? Did they deliberately choose the chair?
- How are they sitting, do they look engaged, are they leaning forward or crouching back in their seat?
- What expression do they have on their face – anger, enthusiasm, disinterest, etc?

As the group begins to meet regularly:

- Has a clique developed, do group members cluster?
- Is there any animosity between group members?
- Are there absences?
- Are any members being isolated?
- Do all members contribute?

Maintaining the group requires attention to the communication within the group and also identification of where the power lies. The Johari Window (Luft, 1970) may be considered when attempting to improve communication. It is comprised of four quadrants (see Figure 7.1). The open area contains behaviours that both self and others are aware of. The deliberately hidden area contains those behaviours known to self but which are hidden from others. The blind quadrant contains behaviours that others are aware of but self is not. This indicates the degree of personal reflection and insight of an individual. The final quadrant contains characteristics that both self and others have yet to discover (Jacques, 1996).

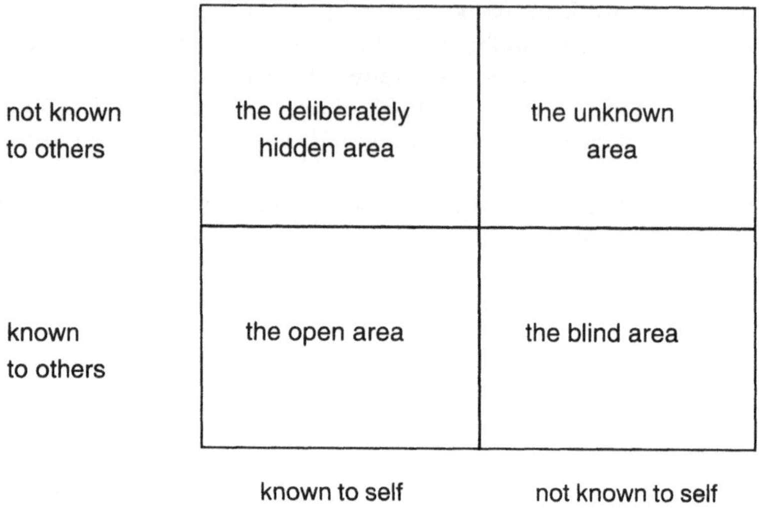

Figure 7.1 The Johari Window

Individuals will have varying degrees of open, hidden, unknown and blind areas. One of the aims of small group work is to expand each participant's open area and in so doing reduce the blind, hidden and unknown area. Moving from a quadrant to a circular depiction the open area can be seen to replace the other aspects (see Figure 7.2) as a means to improve communication.

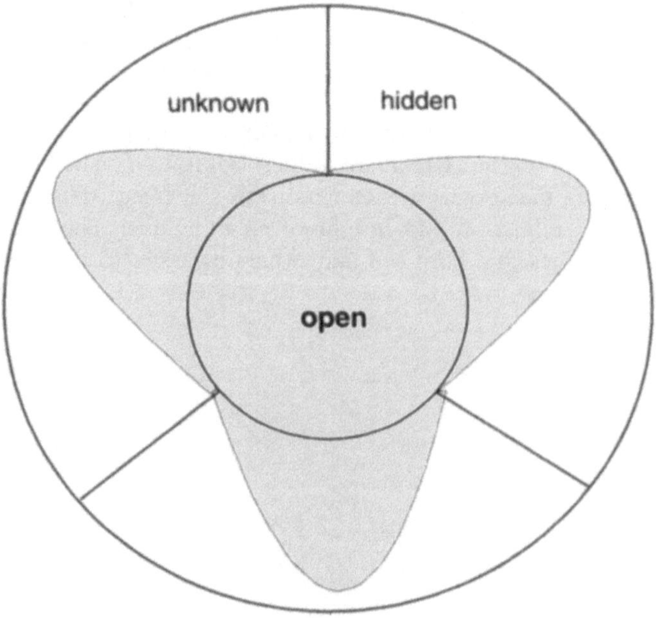

Figure 7.2 Widening the open area in the Johari Window

Who should be a facilitator?

The characteristics of a facilitator are important. Should facilitators be experts in the content the students are learning? Should they be experts in facilitation or experts in both? The research is unequivocal that the facilitator should be familiar with the skills of facilitation (Barrows, 1988). However, it has been suggested that content experts may have a detrimental effect on collaborative learning (Wilkerson, Hafler and Lui, 1991) as they are more likely to talk too long, too often and have a more directive role. Even unwittingly, once students detect expertise there may be a tendency to commit themselves less actively.

However, Davis, Nairn and Anderson (1990), found that students' evaluations of small group work were higher in small groups led by content experts. The need for the facilitator to be both a content expert and good facilitator may vary with the type of small group. In a tutorial an expert is required to identify incorrect material. However, in a free discussion group where opinions may be discussed the requirement is less pressing.

The role of the student as the facilitator should be considered (Crosby, 1996). This may be a member of the group or a slightly more senior student from outside. Peer facilitation has advantages. Students are likely to talk more openly with peers than members of staff. Students as facilitators may also have had experience of learning a topic and therefore are more likely to help by appreciating the difficulty junior students have with certain topics. Peer facilitation is also advantageous as it develops the facilitator skills of the student.

However, students can work and function in a group independently of a facilitator (Crosby, 1996). This more closely replicates informal learning groups in a postgraduate setting. It may be advantageous to have a facilitator present at the start up of a group to keep it on task, but these and maintenance functions may then be given to the students. This may start in a moderate way, for example a student being asked to keep time, to more sophisticated roles, for example, encouraging participation by all. Alternatively, students may like to take it in turns to act as the facilitator. This will help develop facilitatory skills that may be useful in the future.

If the number of available staff is limited, floating facilitators may be considered who move amongst a number of groups. This will affect the dynamics of the group but may be an acceptable alternative.

Coping with small group problems

Sometimes it is difficult to determine the problem within a group. There may not be an easily identifiable cause. If a group is not functioning effectively the facilitator should ask the group what they think the problem is. Sometimes it may be due to lack of clarity regarding the purpose of the group (Tiberius, 1999). Sometimes it may be that they do not value the subject matter, they think the outcomes are unattainable or unacceptable (Tiberius, 1999). These issues need to be carefully addressed as part of the task functions of the facilitator.

Sometimes if a group has been completing work independently of the facilitator, the facilitator may be the problem. The facilitator should leave a group on occasions and observe whether this results in greater communication between the group members. The group may not wish the facilitator to be present. The facilitator should take this rejection with pride, as the group feels able to function independently.

There are obvious types of individual behaviour that may result in the group not performing adequately. There is a danger of suggesting an overall strategy for addressing problem students. Each situation is different and each student and group of students is different. What may work in one situation may fail to work in a similar but subtly different situation. The following are merely simple suggestions for what can be a complex situation, (see Table 7.4). The facilitator may negotiate with a group that at various junctures the dynamics of the group are evaluated. This may allow a frank exchange of opinions regarding the behaviour of group members that may be problematic. Although sometimes tempting, disciplining a problem student whilst in the small group setting is generally unwise. The position of power is immediately altered, taking responsibility away from the group and this may be detrimental to learning. As a last resort, a discussion with the individual separately, and in confidence, to discuss their behaviour may be necessary.

Rather than adopt pre-packaged advice on how to deal with problem group members it is more appropriate for the facilitator to reflect on the situation, act, evaluate any change that has occurred due to the action and consider how that experience may be used to inform future action in a similar situation. Facilitating small groups is an experiential and ongoing learning experience.

Table 7.4 Coping with student small group problems

'The student is ...	Problem	Strategy
'A joker'	In small doses the joker may be very good for the morale of the group. However, if all aspects of the group work or individuals' contributions are ridiculed then it may become tedious and undermine the work of the group.	In the first instance the facilitator should not encourage the behaviour by finding the jokes amusing. If the joker persists then the facilitator should challenge the joker's comments and ask for justification.
'A know it all'	Individuals who express an opinion about everything are problematic as they may inhibit others from contributing.	Ask for specific contributions from other members of the group. Revert back to the 'know it all' when others have contributed.
'An aggressive'	The individual who aggressively challenges everything is disruptive due to the embarrassment it may cause the group and also the often inappropriateness of the questioning.	Do not be drawn into petty arguments. Acknowledge the contribution but do not get distracted from the task at hand.
'Bored'	Boredom is disruptive and detrimental, as it can be contagious.	Try and engage or excite the individual. Try and find out what is boring and also indicate the negative effect it may have on the group members.
'Timid and/or quiet'	The timid/quiet student will contribute infrequently and may appear embarrassed and sometimes apologetic. This group member may be easily dissuaded from an opinion.	An attempt has to be made to ensure that this member contributes in order to check understanding. Direct questioning may be necessary. Be especially supportive of contributions by the timid/quiet individuals. Small groups may well be a useful setting in which the timid individual may become more assertive.
'Absent'	Absenteeism it not only detrimental for the individual but may also antagonize the group who feel that the workload is not evenly spread.	Keep a register – even if mental. Find out the reasons for non-attendance. Address these reasons if possible. Make attendance compulsory. Make attendance a component of assessment. Make peer assessment a component of assessment.

Problem-based learning

What is PBL?

In recent years the value of learning in small groups is no better exemplified than in the movement to problem-based learning (PBL). Much has been written about PBL. PBL is more than just a type of small group method, it is an educational philosophy from which the whole planning of a curriculum stems. The core feature of 'pure' PBL is that students are responsible for determining what they have to learn and then for learning it. PBL is not only student-centred, but also adopts key tenets of adult learning (Brookfield, 1988). Schmidt identifies PBL by three essential principles (Schmidt, 1983):

- **Activation of prior learning** is the starting point for the development of understanding.
- **Encoding specificity**. The specific content and context of the learning produces a type of encoding operation that produces a memory trace that can be readily retrieved in later clinical practice.
- **Elaboration of knowledge**. The small group setting facilitates the elaboration of knowledge, usually through discussion, reflection and consolidation of learning. It is often achieved through social negotiation, testing, re-evaluating and evolving understanding (Savery and Duffy, 1995).

The problem-based learning cycle has been summarized in Figure 7.3. The first key step in problem-based learning is the identification, by students, of what they need to learn. The facilitator should introduce the students to a clinical case. The case may be presented in a written format or as a real, stimulated or videoed patient, but needs to be well prepared in advance of the session.

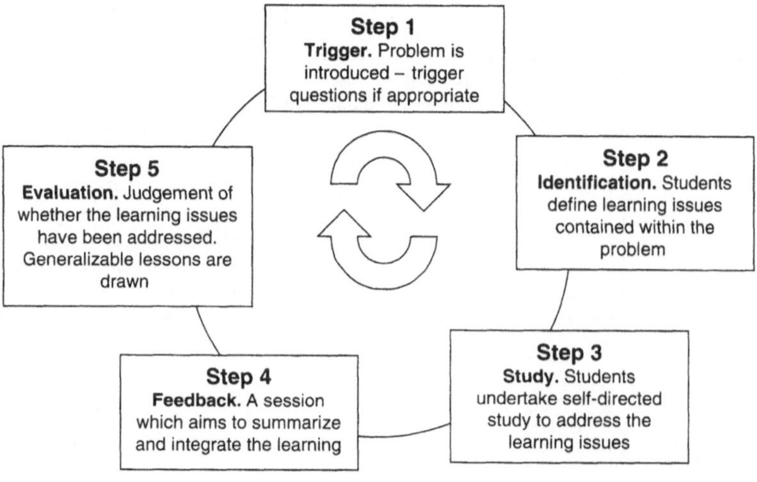

Figure 7.3 Problem-based learning cycle (modified from Elwyn *et al*, 2001)

In the second stage the students have a responsibility to list the learning issues related to the case. At a simple level it may include uncertainty regarding the terminology, and at a more detailed level the potential investigations and management options may be considered. It is important that the underlying basic and clinical sciences are considered in conjunction with any clinical focus. In order to generate the learning issues a brainstorming technique may be advantageous. It is important in the first stage not to discount any issues identified.

The students can then appraise the learning issues. They may wish to group certain issues, discount some or even expand the range of issues. Once a final list of learning issues has been produced the students have to consider a strategy for ensuring that they are all addressed. The strategy may involve the division of work or all the students addressing all of the issues.

Once a strategy has been determined the students are required to conduct research, stage 3, in order to address the issues. The time spent researching the issues depends on the length and complexity of the case and the resources available. It is important that adequate resources are made available to students. This may include library books, clinical opportunities and even 'whole group' sessions in order to clarify difficult concepts. However, all the opportunities on the course should be focussed around the problems given to the students. The problems are the driving force of the curriculum.

Once the research has been conducted the student returns to integrate their learning. This session is stage 4 in the problem-based learning cycle. If students have been given specific aspects to research on their own, this meeting may take the form of a seminar with presentations to the rest of the group. It may be useful to have a content expert at this session.

Finally the students and facilitator evaluate the session. The first part of this stage requires evaluation of how well the learning issues have been addressed. The students should also identify generalizable points from the cases and also what they feel they still need to know.

Generation of case/problem to be used in PBL

'The development of productive, manageable, appropriate learning issues is central to students' achievement of content objectives in problem-based learning' (Quinlan, 2000). The likelihood of learners generating desirable learning objectives is dependent on the quality of the stimulus material given to the students. It requires a good deal of creativity and testing in order to ensure that all criteria are satisfied to prove effective at promoting the desired learning. PBL planners (David *et al*, 1999) should consider the design features in Table 7.5.

Table 7.5 Planning problems for problem-based learning

What is the student's existing knowledge and skills?	In formulating a PBL case the level of the student's prior knowledge and skills should be considered.
Is it relevant?	The problems devised should relate to the core curriculum that is deemed appropriate by the school as covering relevant key issues.
Is it realistic?	Problems should be realistic and not contrived. It is useful to consider actual experiences in formulating questions.[1]
Is it engaging?	PBL cases should enthuse students.[1] Motivation is a key tenet of learning and the cases should be engaging.
Is it set at an appropriate level?	Not only should prior learning be considered but also the stage of education or training for the learner.
Is the problem concise?	Problems that are too long may result in students being distracted from the intended learning issues.[2]
How will this problem influence the learning approach of the student?	In formulating a problem consider whether the problem will encourage students to attend the library, seek out clinical material, discuss and debate, etc.
Are there enough resources for the student to research the problem?	PBL relies on student self-study. Opportunities must be provided for study. This may involve access to patients, written material and/or or plenary sessions to clarify difficult concepts.
Has the student enough time to complete the problem?	Time must be allowed for all stages of the PBL cycle to be completed.

[1] Glick and Armstrong, 1996
[2] David et al, 1999

Types of problems

There are many medical examples of problem cases used in PBL from as early as the early 1970s (Neufeld and Barrows, 1974). The following example asks the learner to explain the phenomena described in terms of underlying processes. Cold Hands (David *et al*, 1999):

> Johnny Green, seven-years-old, is playing bare-handed in the snow on a beautiful clear winter day. After a while, he notices that his hands have become quite cold and look pale. By the time Johnny arrives home crying,

his hands have turned blue. 'My hands are so cold', he tells his mother. Despite Johnny's loud protest, his mother holds his hands under the cold water tap. 'Feeling better?' she asks after a while. 'They are glowing', Johnny replies. 'It feels like a million needles pricking'.

The following is an example from *Veterinary Medicine*. Problem-based scenario (Quinlan, 2000):

A seven-year-old golden retriever is presented with anorexia, incoordination, weakness and icterus. History includes chronic treatment with primidone for seizures. Initial workup indicates increased serum activities of AST, ALT and alkaline phosphatase. Supportive chronic liver disease is rendered. Periodic checkups indicate gradual improvement in liver function. Potassium bromide is used to control seizures with partial success.

With the improvement in information technology some schools use computer software to sequentially display problems. The following Web site is one example in obstetrics: http://www2.onnet.co.kr/ smcobgy/obsteto.html.

Advantages and disadvantages of PBL

Student evaluations indicate that PBL is more enjoyable, relevant, more humane than more traditional didactic methods of learning and also prepares students better to handle uncertainty (Bligh, 1995). Unfortunately, little evidence is available to indicate if PBL is any better at improving academic or clinical performance in comparison with other small group strategies. Comparisons with didactic teaching are considered in Chapter 4.

Staff and PBL

Problem-based learning is not an easy option for a lecturer. The success of the method hinges on appropriate facilitation and high-quality stimulus material. Some schools may find staff reticent to make such a commitment.

A PBL continuum has been proposed, which may encourage MDV Schools to find the incorporation of PBL a feasible option (Davis and Harden, 1998). They suggest that the PBL continuum has theoretical learning at one end and task-based learning at the other. They define two intermediate stages as problem-assisted learning, where information is provided for the student to apply to a clinical problem. This is a more teacher-centred mode of learning. A further intermediate stage is defined as problem-initiated learning where a problem is used to interest the students in the particular topic. Clear reasons for adopting PBL should be considered and the curriculum developed around this key philosophy. Small-scale trials of PBL may be adopted but time is often required for students and staff to understand the philosophy and also to start effectively performing in their groups.

Conclusion

Small group learning is an invaluable method of learning. It is not only useful in developing deep understanding of a topic but in developing personal generic attributes, for example, communication skills, team-working skills, presentation skills and debating skills. In addition, small group work more accurately reflects the adult learning styles that will be adopted in the postgraduate setting. Small group work is not an easy educational method to adopt. It requires forward planning, staff skilled in facilitation and frequently the availability of resource material and space. Small group work should have clear learning outcomes and a number of different small group methods can be adopted to fulfil these outcomes. The role of the facilitator is important and should be understood by all members of the small group. The key tasks of facilitators are to ensure that the students complete the learning outcomes associated with the small group work and maintain the cohesion of the group, which makes this possible.

Problem-based learning encapsulates all the key features of small group work and the facilitation of learning. It is an educational approach usually centred around clinical problems. What distinguishes and elevates it from other methods of learning is the requirement of the learner to identify their own learning issues and to encourage students to take responsibility for their own learning. Small group work is advocated as a valuable method of learning that should be adopted in some format in the MDV undergraduate curriculum.

References

Barrows, H S (1988) *The Tutorial Process*, Southern Illinois University School of Medicine, Springfield, IL

Bion, W (1961) *Experiences in groups*, Tavistock, London

Bligh, J (1995) Problem-based, small group learning, *British Medical Journal*, **311**, pp 342–43

Brookfield, S D (1988) *Understanding and facilitating adult learning*, OUP, Buckingham

Cox, K R and Ewan, C E (1988) *The Medical Teacher*, Churchill Livingstone, Edinburgh

Crosby, J (1996) Learning in Small Groups, *Medical Teacher*, **18** (3), pp 189–202

David, T *et al* (1999) *Problem-based learning in Medicine*, The Royal Society of Medicine Books, London

Davis, M H and Harden, R M (1998) The continuum of problem based learning, *Medical Teacher*, **20**, pp 317–22

Davis, W K, Nairn, R and Anderson, R M (1990) Effects of experts and non-expert facilitation on the small group process and on student performance, *Academic Medicine*, **67**, pp 470–74

Elwyn, G, Greenhalgh, T and MacFarlen, F (2001) *Groups: a guide to small group work in healthcare, management, education and research*, Radcliffe Medical Press Ltd, Oxford

Entwistle, N, Thompson, S and Tait, H (1992) *Guide for promoting effective learning in higher education*, Centre for Research on Learning and Instruction, Edinburgh

Glick, T H and Armstrong, E G (1996) Crafting cases for problem-based learning: experience in a neuroscience course, *Medical Education*, **30**, pp 24–30

Harden, R M, Sowden, S and Dunn, W R (1984) *Some Educational Strategies in Curriculum Development: The SPICES Model*, Medical Education Booklet edn v, 18, ASME, Edinburgh

Honey, P and Mumford, A (1982) *The Manual of Learning Styles*, Peter Honey, Maidenhead

Jacques, D (1996) *Learning in small groups*, Kogan Page, London

Kolb, D A (1984) *Experiential learning experience as the source of learning and development*, Prentice-Hall, Englewood Cliffs

Luft, J (1970) *Group processes: an introduction to group dynamics*, National Press Books, Pal Antonio, California

McKeachie, W J (1986) *Teaching tips: a guidebook for the beginning college teacher*, 8th edn, D C Heath and Co, Lexington, Mass

McLeod, P J and Harden, R M (1985) Clinical teaching strategies for physicians, *Medical Teacher*, **72**, pp 173–89

Neufield, V and Barrows, H (1974) The 'McMaster philosophy': an approach to medical education, *Journal of Medical Education*, **49**, pp 1040–50

Quinlan, K M (2000) *Generating productive learning issues in PBL: an exercise to help tutors help students*, [Online] http://www:med-ed-online.org http://www:med-ed-online.org

Raaheim, K (1991) On the pedagogical skills of university teachers, in *Helping students to learn: teaching, counselling, research*, ed K Raaheim, Open University Press, Buckingham

Renzulli, J S and Smith, L H *et al* (2002) *Scales for Rating the Behavioral Characteristics of Superior Students: Technical and Administration Manual* (revised edn), Creative Learning Press, Mansfield Center, CT

Savery, J R and Duffy, T M (1995) Problem based learning: an instructional model and its constructivism framework, *Education Technology*, **35** (5), pp 31–38

Schmidt, H G (1983) Problem-based learning: rationale and description, *Medical Education*, **17** (1), pp, 11–16

Springer, L, Stanne, M E and Donovan, S S (1999) Effects or small group learning on undergraduates in science, mathematics, engineering and technology: a meta analysis, *Review of Educational Research*, **69**, pp 21–51

Thelen, H and Dickerman, W (1949) Stereotypes and the growth of groups, *Educational Leadership*, **6**, pp 309–16

Tiberius, R G (1999) *Small group teaching: a trouble-shooting guide*, Kogan Page, London

Tuckman, B W (1965) Development sequence in small groups, *Psychological Bulletin*, **63**, pp 384–99

Tuckman, B W and Jensen, M A (1977) Stages of small group development, *Group and organisational studies*, **2**, p 4

Vernon, D T and Blake, R L (1993) Does problem-based learning work? A meta-analysis of evaluative research, *Academic Medicine*, **68** (7), pp 550–63

Walton, H J (1997) Small Group Methods in Medical Teaching, *Medical Education*, **31**, pp 457–64

Wilkerson, L, Hafler, J P and Lui, P (1991) A case study of student-directed discussion in four problem-based tutorial groups, *Academic Medicine*, **66** (9), pp S79–S81

8

Using information technologies and teaching online

John Eyers and Andrew Sackville

Introduction

One of the greatest challenges for all tutors in recent years has been attempting to keep abreast of the accelerating pace of technological change and developments. Government reports in both the United Kingdom and the United States have singled out the spread of the Internet as the most rapid technological development we have ever experienced (easily outstripping the introduction of radio and television) (for example, see US Congress, 2000). We have seen computers shrink in size, become more affordable and more reliable; and it is clear that this trend is not going to stop. Gilbert (2000) has argued that the safest prediction is that 'in the next decade at least one major new trend in the educational use of information technology will not have been predicted by anyone highly respected in fields closely related to education or technology'. Already some US universities ensure that all their students and staff have laptops they can plug into the university network wherever they are, and at all times of day and night; whilst a few pioneering universities are experimenting with 'wireless' computers, using radio waves on a campus, allowing even more flexibility. There clearly remain a number of technical problems about the reliability of systems, and ensuring equality of access to the technology is an issue. But, as William Gibson, the inventor of the term 'cyberspace', has stated: 'The future is here. It is just not evenly distributed' (Gibson, 1999).

As important as the developing technology itself, is the permeation of that technology into our daily working practices. Communications and information technology (C&IT) has increasingly permeated most aspects of professional activity in medical, dental and veterinary (MDV) practice – the use of extensive databases, the updating of records and information, the linking with fellow professionals via a video-conference. Similarly C&IT is influencing MDV education at all levels – undergraduate, postgraduate and continuing professional development. Our graduates need to be comfortable in this new computer-mediated environment, and they need to be able to adapt to developments in knowledge and the pace of technological change by being lifelong learners. Educators have a responsibility to help prepare graduates for this aspect of professional practice.

There is of course a danger of being caught up in the accompanying hype of some of these technological developments; but as educators we need to grasp the opportunities presented by technological change, to recognize and harness the strengths of the technology to support our teaching and the students' learning, and to be aware of the limitations of the technology. C&IT must be conceived as a tool that can enhance learning – not as an end in itself. It is this belief that informs this chapter.

The chapter begins by discussing some of the general issues of relating C&IT to teaching and learning, before moving on to focus on two major aspects of working with electronic information and engaging in electronic communication. These two aspects are then combined to analyse the ways in which C&IT has been used in MDV education. Some examples of the use of C&IT are described, before the chapter concludes by examining ways in which tutors can start using C&IT, or can use C&IT more effectively in their teaching and learning facilitation.

General issues of C&IT in education

There are many terms and acronyms for using technology in education – for example IT, ICT, CME, CBL, etc. Some terms tend to be historic, whilst others relate to specific applications of technology – but we are using the term communications and information technology (C&IT) in this chapter. For us the phrase C&IT symbolizes the importance of the interaction between communications, information and technology. The accessing and use of information, and engagement in various forms of communication, has always been of critical importance in professional education and professional practice, but the use of technology brings the skills of effectively using information and communication into sharper relief.

The application of C&IT to MDV education has extended over a number of years (for some early examples see Leicester University, 1994). Many pioneering projects have explored the application of different aspects of the technology to MDV education, but in recent years there has been a groundswell of institutions jumping on the C&IT bandwagon, particularly linked to the development of the Internet and campus networks (Ward *et al*, 2001).

We would argue that C&IT should not be an add-on in any learning and teaching experience, but it should be planned and integrated within the curriculum, whether at undergraduate, postgraduate or CPD level. As Goodyear (2001) has argued, this will often mean going back to first principles in designing the curriculum, and in planning learning and teaching activities. Course planners have always had to address the questions – how do our students learn and how can we support and help develop that learning? And what sort of learning do we want to encourage – active, problem-based, evidence-based, collaborative learning? In addition, course planners now need to add the dimension of mode of delivery to their planning questions – will the teaching be face-to-face, online, at a distance? What are the most appropriate methods of delivery?

It would be easy to use computers simply as a means of delivering one-way information to students (as the traditional model of the lecture or textbook does), but the technology now available allows tutors to explore and use a number of different dimensions of interactivity, which will support and reinforce students in their active learning. We would suggest that there are at least five dimensions of interactivity that need to be built into the planning and development stage of the curriculum:

- Firstly there is the interaction between the students and the technology to be used in their learning. Students must feel comfortable with the technology, whether it is a CAL package or the use of the World Wide Web.
- Secondly there is the need to plan for interaction between the students and the information/content that they are studying. It is all too easy to simply present students with information or content, and then expect them to 'work' on it. The use of technology makes the course developer ask how we want the students to use the content/information, and how we can encourage this effective use.
- Thirdly there is the interaction between student and tutor. How will this be arranged – one-to-one, in small groups, as a total group? When will the interaction take place – on demand, at set times, synchronously or asynchronously?
- Fourthly if we are wishing to encourage collaborative learning, and the development of the skills of working in groups, the designer has to consider the interaction between students themselves. How do we encourage them to work in groups?
- Finally there is the interaction between the students and their wider professional community. C&IT allows for much greater involvement in this form of interaction than traditional teaching methods. Links can be made into professional practice and into professional expertise worldwide.

The planner and developer roles become increasingly overt when much of the programme is available electronically for students. Very often the material and the interactions between students and tutors are open to external scrutiny, and they are also preserved for the life of the programme – the 'secret classroom' is opened up.

Working with electronic information

Much has been written over the last few decades about the information explosion in print material and attempts to control the burgeoning literature, but the advent of electronic information and its availability over the Internet, in particular, has made more urgent the need for better skills in information searching and evaluation among MDV students, whether undergraduate or postgraduate. Increasingly, the full range of information resources is being made available electronically whether it be journals, databases (such as Medline, Cochrane Library, Embase), textbooks, course handouts, as well as other important resources such as discussion group Web sites and subject-based speciality Web sites. It could now be argued that the main vehicle for MDV information and research is de facto electronic or Web-based. What is generally acknowledged is that the development of electronic MDV information will increase and will become the student's (and ultimately the qualified professional's) first port of call for information, even though this will not eliminate the need for print or library resources.

Most MDV curricula include some form of information skills training, but this training is often divorced from subject teaching and the skills acquired are seen more as transferable skills, since much of this teaching is carried out by librarians and information specialists, who may be perceived as ancillary to the main teaching process. This perception is not often lost on the students themselves who may consider such sessions peripheral to their studies, and consequently pay less attention to the importance of information skills. Often sessions are scheduled at the beginning of courses during the orientation or induction period, a period when students are not fully engaged in their course. The result is that when students do need to use their information skills, they may well have forgotten much of what they learnt earlier, if indeed any effective learning took place at all!

The little evidence that exists as to the way students access information using C&IT suggests that they will use it on a 'need to know' or 'just in time learning' approach at a time when course assignments are due. This will invariably result in less effective information retrieval (Greenhalgh, 2001). The reason for this may be that the time needed to become proficient in using these resources is often underestimated and not sufficient time is devoted to training. Students will thus put off such an investment in time taken to learn the skills until they need to and most may get by in the meantime by relying on more conventional sources such as textbooks and other print material derived from reading lists. One study, which investigated student use of electronic resources, found that large numbers of students were 'leaving university without the necessary transferable skills to cope in an information based society' (Ray and Day, 1998).

However, as more MDV courses become problem- and evidence-based, with a greater dependency on accessing information through C&IT, so the need to integrate fully the information skills component of the curriculum into mainstream teaching becomes crucial. Since information handling skills (searching, selecting, evaluating) are such an essential component of the evidence-based approach, more sophisticated skills are needed in database searching, selecting and critically evaluating articles and in searching the Internet more effectively and critically.

Part of this must also include training to critically assess the quality, validity and currency of the source itself, since there is often an uncritical acceptance of databases, the Internet and other resources when this may not be justified. Medline, for example, may be excellent for clinical and laboratory medicine, but other databases may be better for desk-based health research. All of this sends a clear message that information skills are an important feature of course work. Anecdotal evidence in which this integrated approach has been used at postgraduate taught course level at the London School of Hygiene and Tropical Medicine suggests that students quickly become familiar and adept at using appropriate electronic sources when it is tied into the curriculum itself and more particularly when the work in hand is assessed. Routine use of these resources thus becomes second nature to any information gathering whether for class work, seminars or written work.

What, then, are the essential components of information skills training? The Standing Conference on National and University Libraries (SCONUL) has identified the following as essential to achieve 'information literacy' (SCONUL, 1999):

- the ability to recognize a need for information;
- the ability to distinguish ways in which the information may be addressed:
  - knowledge of appropriate sources;
  - selection of resources for task in hand;
  - ability to understand the issues affecting accessibility of resources;
- the ability to construct strategies for locating information;
- the ability to locate and access information:
  - to develop appropriate search techniques (eg use of Boolean operators);
  - to use C&IT
  - to use indexing/abstracting services, citation indexes and databases;
  - to use current awareness methods to keep up to date;
- the ability to compare and evaluate information obtained from different sources:
  - awareness of bias and authority issues;
  - awareness of the peer review process;
  - appropriate extracting of information matching the information need;
- the ability to organize, apply and communicate information to others in ways appropriate to the situation:
  - to cite correctly bibliographic references in project reports and theses;
  - to construct a personal bibliographic system;
  - to apply information selected;
  - to communicate effectively using an appropriate medium;
  - to understand copyright and plagiarism issues;
- the ability to synthesize and build upon existing information, contributing to the creation of new knowledge.

Who should teach these skills? There is a view that it should be the subject tutors themselves, since they are close to and familiar with the discipline. However, many HE institutions have accepted that, since most subject tutors themselves may lack the necessary information skills associated with using the technologies, librarians and other information specialists are better able to fulfil the role, a view endorsed by HEFCE, which sponsored teaching courses for librarians (such as the Edulib scheme). However, collaboration with discipline experts is essential for designing innovative exercises in information handling that foster information literacy.

Engaging in electronic communication

One of the first and ubiquitous uses of technology for communicating was the development of e-mail. Few professional practitioners are not using e-mail in some way. Some educational institutions use it to such an extent that when there is a systems fault and e-mail is not available – work almost grinds to a halt!

The use of e-mail is not without some limitations. Text-based messages may not have the expressive richness of a quick and lively verbal exchange; there may be less immediacy; levels of discourse may be at odds; and not everyone takes to communication through irregular short text messages (Goodyear, 2001). However, many course programme designers who build electronic communication into their programmes do recognize these limitations but argue that the advantages of greater ease of access between students and between tutors and students, the encouragement of an element of reflection into the communication process (often missing in face-to-face conversations), and the active engagement of students using e-mail, more than compensate for the disadvantages.

The advent of the World Wide Web allowed groups of individuals sharing a common interest to set up Web discussion groups. Dealt with by listservers, these groups may permit open access to all interested parties, or they may be limited to a closed list of participants. They usually use asynchronous discussion – allowing for ideas to be collaboratively developed, information exchanged and innovative practice to be shared. Tutors can set up similar listserve groups for their own students; or can link them into national groups of one kind or another.

A development from the simple use of e-mail was the establishment of conferencing systems (such as FirstClass), where groups of students and tutors are linked together. These conference systems first developed in distance education, but latterly the potential for using conferencing systems with students on campuses has been recognized. Conferencing systems can be used synchronously (often called 'chat rooms') where students and tutors are all online at the same time; or they may be used asynchronously, where the discussion on a topic may be scheduled over a week or a similar period of time.

In planning to use a conferencing system, course developers need to consider how to handle the social interaction that takes place alongside the academic discourse. Some designers have experimented with having separate 'common-rooms' – chat rooms for students, from which tutors are excluded. Our own experience has been that students will incorporate social interaction into their academic interaction, and they are able to 'police' the interactions themselves, without the tutors intervening.

Some tutors have experimented with the use of video-conferencing as a way of enhancing the richness of C&IT communications between students and tutors. Video-conferencing has been used for distance-based students; and it has been used to bring remotely-based subject 'experts' into the classroom. A variant – interactive television – is extensively used in the United States, although it has had less impact in the United Kingdom.

These various communication tools were initially developed separately from the electronic information tools (discussed above) but perhaps the most significant development of the last 10 years has been the bringing together of information and communications into what are often called virtual learning environments (VLEs).

Some higher education institutions have been developing their own VLEs, but most have been adopting existing commercial VLE packages (such as WebCT and Blackboard). These VLEs allow a programme designer to choose to combine a series of applications and tools into a single Web site. Thus electronic information about the programme can be combined with access to information in electronic journals or Web pages; and set alongside communication tools such as e-mail and a conferencing system. This provides ease of access not only for students, but for tutors as well.

VLEs are also allowing tutors to incorporate audio and video material alongside the more frequently used text-based material. A very rich package combining both information and communications can be designed for students.

Combining information, communications and technology for teaching

The technological developments in electronic information and communications outlined above, allow us to design course programmes to promote specific approaches to learning and teaching that can be delivered or supported online. For example, problem-based learning can be supported online. Using a VLE it is possible to present the initial problem scenario (whether specifically written or a 'real-life' event) online. The small groups, with their facilitator, can then explore the scenario using electronic communication; searches for electronic material can be made in databases and electronic journals; the groups can synthesize their knowledge and research data in electronic format; they may use associated electronic concept-mapping tools; and the hypotheses can be evaluated online (see Rendas *et al*, 1999; Rideout, 2001).

Similarly, collaborative learning and active learning, and skills such as discussion, analysis, and critical thinking can be built into the design of materials and activities presented in a VLE (see Bonk and Reynolds, 1997; Baker and Lund, 1997; Gold, 2001).

Online teaching and learning facilitation might be conceived as only appealing to students with certain learning styles, but our experience of online teaching suggests that a carefully designed programme using a VLE with multiple functions can meet the learning needs of students with a variety of learning styles. They can select the material that is most appropriate to themselves (O'Connor, no date). In addition, research has been completed on issues of 'non-participation' in online programmes, or witness learning as it is sometimes called in the United States (Hammond, 1999; McKenzie and Murphy, 2000).

But such examples of online programmes are at one end of a continuum. Programmes can be supported by using networked facilities in a number of other ways. For example, some courses may simply have a Web presence – where minimal information about the programme is online and where e-mail or notice-boards may be used for one-way communication with students. Some programmes may be Web-supported or Web-enhanced; where some of the content, and links to electronic resources are on the Web. But a qualitative leap takes place when it is decided to use the Web to 'teach' – when a Web-centric course is designed. Here the communication element between tutors and students, and between students themselves comes to the fore. The Web material is deliberately designed to be interactive. In reaching the decision as to which model to pursue, the key for the tutor is to decide whether the technology is being used appropriately to support student learning (see Greenhalgh, 2001).

The examples given above have focussed on the use of the Internet and the Web; but many computer programs have been developed as stand-alone packages. There are many examples of such packages in MDV education. One of the best-known projects is the CLIVE Project (Computer-aided Learning in Veterinary Education), which has produced a range of electronic materials for use in both undergraduate teaching and professional development (CLIVE, 2001). These packages have received a mixed evaluation from users – but often this may be linked to how they have been used, rather than to the quality of the contents. Multimedia packages certainly have a role in teaching specific topics or skills in part of the MDV curriculum – but they need to be integrated with the overall educational approach of the learning programme of which they are a part (Greenhalgh, 2001).

The use of VLEs also allows some aspects of assessment, particularly the use of quizzes and multiple-choice questions, to be integrated into the learning environment. Alternatively specialist assessment software packages have been developed. This is a complex topic, which is still being investigated by tutors, and interested readers are referred to other standard texts on the topic (Brown, Bull and Race, 1999; Maier and Warren, 2000).

Examples of the use of C&IT in MDV education

Increasingly, accounts of how specific learning programmes are using C&IT and online teaching are appearing in print, or on the Web. These are useful materials for colleagues who are considering using C&IT in their own teaching. The Faculty of Medicine and Medical Sciences in the University of Aberdeen has presented a case study of how it has developed CAL and other IT resources in the undergraduate medical curriculum (Hamilton *et al*, 1999). This faculty developed a wide spectrum of CAL applications including learning guides, computer-aided assessment, multimedia tutorials and a suite of patient simulations, which they termed Model Patients. These Model Patients were a series of multimedia patient simulations that could present a different level of content according to the student's level of study. The applications allowed students to explore patient history-taking, investigation, diagnosis, treatment and other aspects of patient management.

In contrast, Edge Hill and Chester Colleges, in association with the Mersey Deanery for Postgraduate Medical and Dental Education, have developed a postgraduate certificate in teaching and learning in clinical practice for professionals in practice who have a significant element of their time devoted to the training and supervision of students and junior professionals. This programme was developed to meet the training needs of a range of senior health professionals who would have difficulty in meeting at a set time each week in one location. Online delivery offered flexibility in time and space; but it also offered the potential of bringing teaching staff from three institutions together, and accessing other expertise internationally via the Internet. In addition online delivery allowed content and information to be modified almost daily – in contrast to perhaps a year's delay in altering print-based materials.

The course planning team shared a concern about how rapidly to move into online learning and they formed a particular conception of 'supported online learning'. This involved a number of features designed to support participants. There were five face-to-face days incorporated in the year-long programme. These sessions helped to create a climate of trust between participants, and enabled tutors to deliver parts of the programme where face-to-face contact was more appropriate for the content matter. The participants were each allocated a personal tutor with whom they could communicate via e-mail, phone, letter, fax, personal visit – whatever suited them best. The decision was made early on in the planning process to adopt a 'set text', which could be referred to within the Web pages that were to be constructed. The virtual learning environment adopted was WebCT and icons were specifically designed for the programme.

This home page allowed students to access specially authored material, which was combined with selected Internet links and electronic journals, communication tools and technical/presentational tools in a single location. The modules on the programme covered topics such as how students learn; assessment and evaluation;

and methods of teaching and learning facilitation. At the same time a series of online activities allowed the participants to reflect on their own experience and to relate this to their colleagues' experiences and to the research and theoretical literature.

The course team had a particular approach to education and a set of professional values that they shared with participants (see Sackville, 2000). They also shared their perceptions of the roles of a tutor on an online programme. These roles included:

- providing and structuring opportunities for participants to reflect on their own and others' practice;
- supporting participants in analysing and exploring their own practice in the context of the theoretical and practical literature;
- exploring implicit theories of teaching, learning and assessment, and making these explicit;
- identifying a corpus of knowledge that participants could access and evaluate;
- offering signposts to the study of specific topics;
- helping participants identify skills that they may wish to develop further;
- running and encouraging asynchronous online discussions and seminars;
- responding to participants' individual concerns and interest;
- modelling/demonstrating different forms of teaching and learning facilitation;
- assessing the completed products of the assessment process and recommending the award of the qualification.

Ongoing evaluation of the programme has been positive, although the programme team made certain modifications between the first two presentations of the programme to support participants in gaining confidence in their interaction with the technology. The tutors found that the introduction of a two-and-a-half-week mini-module on using the technology to assist in study and communication, before the introduction of the first content module, certainly enhanced the appropriate use of the technology by the second cohort. The evidence from the first cohort demonstrated that the 20 successful participants used the technology in different ways to support their own learning, but the sense of being a cohesive learning community of students and tutors was very strong. Further analysis of the contribution of participants to the online discussion is continuing; and this is in turn leading to modifications in some of the online activities – to encourage even greater participation.

The online tutors have had to learn new skills in facilitating online activities, but the experience has been both challenging and exhilarating. It must however be stressed that the programme team designed the programme from clear pedagogic principles, involving both active and reflective learning, based on a social constructivist model of learning. The technology was used to support this approach. Technology did not drive the programme; it simply allowed access for busy professionals to a learning community, which was not constrained by time or place, and which supported those individuals and interest groups in their own professional development as teachers – an opportunity that would have been lost without the effective use of C&IT.

Using C&IT effectively

It is easy to be somewhat overwhelmed by the possibilities of using C&IT in your teaching and learning facilitation. But there are many forms of assistance now available to those who wish to incorporate C&IT into their programmes.

There are an increasing number of introductory texts (written in non-technical language, and written from a pedagogic rather than a technical perspective). Some are available in print, some online; and increasingly print-based material has a Web site that can be accessed to support the book (see Salmon, 2000; Maier and Warren, 2000). A number of online publications have arisen from centrally funded initiatives and their material is freely available for use (see particularly Goodyear, 2001; TALENT, 2000; OTIS, 2001).

These core texts can be supplemented by material available on the Internet in various academic institutions worldwide. Among sites that make such links are the University of Oregon (Oregon, 2001); New Brunswick (New Brunswick, 2001) and Ontario (Learn Ontario, 2001).

But these text-based references can be supplemented by contacting and working alongside existing users of C&IT in higher education. We have found the community of C&IT developers to be extremely helpful to new starters with a genuine interest in developing their own practice, whether in their own particular subject or in broader more generic areas of teaching and learning. Annual conferences of professional associations and generic groups such as the Institute for Learning and Teaching (ILT) or the Association for Learning Technology (ALT) in the United Kingdom, provide showcase presentations of cutting edge developments in the use of C&IT. The Learning and Teaching Support Network (LTSN) for MDV education is another source of information on the use of C&IT (see the list of URLs at the conclusion of this chapter).

Because of the range of skills needed in developing C&IT supported programmes, this is an area where lecturers have to work alongside a range of other professionals including resource managers' learning technology designers and technical support staff. For example, the team for developing the post-graduate diploma discussed above comprised four academics, a learning resources manager, a researcher, a learning technology designer, a Web-master, and a technician. There are new skills to be learnt, or old skills to be updated for all involved in developing CAL and online learning. One feature we have noted in developing programmes has been the reduction in isolation of the single academic and the creativity generated by teamwork in a multi-professional team.

As programmes are developed, it is essential to build evaluation into the process, since up to the present time, there has been little evidence of the positive or negative effects of using C&IT in teaching and learning. Greenhalgh (2001) has collected what evidence there is in her article, but many other evaluation studies have yet to be published.

Conclusion

This chapter has demonstrated the enormous potential of integrating C&IT into teaching and learning, but it has also argued the need to incorporate decisions about the appropriate use of technology into the planning and development stages of curriculum design. It has suggested that if we are going to teach and facilitate learning with C&IT this has to be linked to broader ideas about the aims and purposes of teaching; and to a re-evaluation of the role of tutor. Information and communications must be interwoven into any programme design and staff must reflect on the new skills they need to develop to both design and to deliver programmes using C&IT.

References

Baker, M and Lund, K (1997) Promoting reflective interactions in a CSCL environment, *Journal of Computer Assisted Learning*, **13**, pp 177–93

Bonk, C and Reynolds, T (1997) Learner-Centered Web Instruction for Higher-Order Thinking, Teamwork, and Apprenticeship, in *Web-Based Instruction*, ed B H Khan, Educational Technology Publications, New Jersey

Brown, S, Bull, J and Race, P (1999) *Computer Assisted Assessment in Higher Education*, Kogan Page, London

CLIVE – Computer Aided Learning in Veterinary Education (2001) [accessed May 2001] *Home Page* [Online] http://www.clive.ed.ac.uk/

Gibson, W (1999) quoted in Boettcher, J (1999) [accessed May 2001] *21st Century Teaching and Learning Patterns* [Online] http://www.syllabus.com/syllabusmagazine/Jun99_magfea.html

Gilbert, S (2000) [accessed May 2001] Teaching, Learning and Technology Predictions, *LIZARD 52, University of Oregon* [Online] http://darkwing.uoregon.edu/ tep/

Gold, S (2001) A constructivist approach to online training for online teachers, *JALN*, **5** (1), pp 35–57

Goodyear, P (2001) [accessed May 2001] Effective networked learning in higher education: notes and guidelines, *CSALT Lancaster University* [Online] http://csalt.lancs.ac.uk/jisc/advice.htm

Greenhalgh, T (2001) Computer assisted learning in undergraduate medical education, *British Medical Journal*, **322** pp 40–44

Hamilton, N, Furnace, J, Duguid, K, Helms, P and Simpson, J (1999) Development and integration of CAL: a case study in medicine, *Medical Education*, **33**, pp 298–305

Hammond, M (1999) Issues associated with participation in online forums – the case of the communicative learner, *Education and Information Technologies*, **4** (4), pp 353–67

Learn Ontario (2001) [accessed May 2001] *Instructional Design for the New Media* [Online] http://www.rcc.ryerson.ca/learnontario/idnm/frame.htm

Leicester University (1994) Developments in Medical Education, *Enterprise Bibliography No 18*, University of Leicester

LTSN Learning and Teaching Support Network (2001) [accessed May 2001] *Home Page for Medicine, Dentistry and Veterinary Medicine* [Online] http://www.ltsn-01.ac.uk

Maier, P and Warren, A (2000) *Integrating Technology in Learning and Teaching*, Kogan Page, London

McKenzie, W and Murphy, D (2000) 'I hope this goes somewhere': Evaluation of an online discussion group, *Australian Journal of Educational Technology*, **16** (3), pp 239–57

New Brunswick (2001) [accessed May 2001] Learning on the Web, *New Brunswick Distance Education Inc* [Online] http://teleeducation.nb.ca/content/lotw97/

O'Connor, T (no date) [accessed May 2001] *Using Learning Styles to Adapt Technology to Higher Education* [Online] http://Web.indstate.edu/ctl/styles/learning.html

Oregon (2001) [accessed May 2001] Teaching with Technology, *University of Oregon* [Online] http://www.uoregon.edu/ tep/technology/

OTIS Online Tutoring Skills Project (2001) [accessed May 2001] *Online Tutoring e-Book* [Online] http://otis.scotcit.ac.uk/onlinebook/

Ray, K and Day, J (1998) Student attitudes towards electronic information resources, *Information Research*, **4** (2)

Rendas, A, Rosado Pinto, P and Gamboa, T (1999) A computer simulation designed for problem-based learning, *Medical Education*, **33**, pp 47–54

Rideout, E (2001) *Transforming Nursing Education Through Problem-Based Learning*, Jones and Bartlett, Sudbury, Mass

Sackville, A (2000) [accessed May 2001] *Asynchronous Online Learning – a case study* [Online] http://www.edgehill.ac.uk/tld/clinstudy.htm

Salmon, G (2000) *E-Moderating*, Kogan Page, London

SCONUL (Standing Conference on National and University Libraries) (1999) [accessed May 2001] Information Skills in Higher Education; A SCONUL position paper, London [Online] http://www.sconul.ac.uk/publications/99104Revl.doc

TALENT Teaching and Learning using Network Technologies (2001) [accessed May 2001] *The Book of TALENT* [Online] http://www.le.ac.uk/TALENT/book/sitemap.htm

US Congress (2000) [accessed May 2001] *Web-based Education Commission's Final Report* [Online] http://www.Webcommission.org

Ward, J, Gordon, J, Field, M and Lehmann, H (2001) Communication and information technology in medical education, *The Lancet*, **357**, pp 792–96

Useful URLs for further reference

(Please note URLs may change. If these addresses are no longer valid, use a search engine to find the new address.)

URLs on generic aspects of C&IT in teaching and learning

Learning and Teaching Support Network for MDV education
http://www.ltsn-01.ac.uk

Association for Learning Technology
http://www.warwick.ac.uk/alt-E/

Institute for Learning and Teaching in Higher Education
http://www.ilt.ac.uk
Asynchronous Learning Networks (USA)
http://www.aln.org

DeLiberations
http://www.lgu.ac.uk/deliberations

URLs on MDV gateways to electronic information or C&IT initiatives
OMNI Internet Resources for Medical and Biosciences
http://omni.ac.uk

Medical matrix: guide to Internet resources
http://www.medmatrix.org

WISDOM Centre
http://www.shef.ac.uk/uni/projects/wrp/

DERWeb
http://www.derWeb.co.uk

Vetgate
http://vetgate.ac.uk/

Animal health Information Specialists
http://www.ahis.org/

Free Medical Journals Site
http://www.freemedicaljournals.com/fp/go.cfm

9

Supporting students

Jeff Wilson and John Sweet

Introduction

A school leaver achieving high grades at A level has been the traditional student admitted into MDV education, but admission is influenced by the number of places on offer and the demand for those places. Demand has always exceeded supply (many times over), for medicine and veterinary courses, and most of the time for dentistry, although demand declined in the early 1980s in both Sweden (Sjostrom, 1995) and the United Kingdom (Duguid, 1989). In future, Medical Schools in Britain may find themselves competing for the pool of suitable candidates as the government aims to double the number of doctors by widening both access and diversity (see Chapter 14).

At school, students receive mainly didactic teaching and are not prepared for the transition to self-directed learning. Despite an apparent shift in emphasis away from assessment by formal examinations towards continuous assessment of course work, there are constant external pressures on schools to achieve higher grades. Together with tighter control over curriculum content this probably results in students being more spoon-fed and results-driven than ever before.

Traditionally, undergraduate 'freshers' have gone up to university to read their chosen subject. Students in higher education are expected to learn rather than to be taught. This difference can be disconcerting for the majority of school leavers who choose to go straight to university. Undergraduates no longer find themselves being shepherded in their studies. The majority manage to make the transition successfully but there is a broad spectrum of responses to this newly found freedom. Some thoroughly enjoy their first year, only to struggle at the end-of-year examinations. Others work excessively hard only to exhaust themselves.

For many it is also the first time they have left the care and supporting environment of their family home. They are at an age where, although legally adults, they are rapidly finding out about life as an independent individual. Socially, emotionally, sexually, financially and morally they have to start fending for themselves, to rapidly mature as adults. They are also potentially isolated, homesick, worried and vulnerable.

The authors believe that student support, until now initiated at university level, should be extended to start with pre-entry students. They can be encouraged in their work towards entry qualifications and their preparations for university and college admissions service applications. Both Sheffield and Cardiff have started 'compact' schemes for which pupils in previously under-represented areas can register. In Cardiff, student mentors and a 'widening access coordinator' will keep in touch with these students both at school and at a three-day residential summer school. Students will be encouraged to work consistently to achieve at least the minimum entry qualifications for the clinical course and to develop a personal profile that demonstrates communication and team-working skills.

Students have the right to expect to be fully supported by their chosen university. Universities owe a duty of care to their students. They should provide adequate facilities and support to enable students to successfully complete their course of study. Where should new undergraduates find guidance and support?

Supporting undergraduate students

The registry

Having been offered a place and satisfied the entry requirements, students' initial contact with their university will be via the registry. Here they will register as a student, agree to abide by the university rules and regulations, satisfy the financial requirements and proceed to their course of study. In return, the registry should provide all the necessary information to enable students to follow their chosen course. The university has then entered into a contract with each student. In addition to providing an education, it also has a duty of care to students for their continuing welfare throughout the course.

There follows an induction when students are introduced to their faculty and relevant staff. This usually coincides with freshers' week where social events are organized by student unions to enable new students to meet fellow students and staff, familiarize themselves with the various facilities the university has to offer and join various clubs and societies. Freshers' week is an important event as it gives all new students the chance to adapt to their new environment, discover what facilities are available both within the college and locally, and informally discuss with staff and senior students what they are likely to encounter in the coming term. It helps new students begin the process of developing their identity as an undergraduate member of the university.

Financial arrangements are important for the new undergraduate. Most will need to apply for student loans. There may be tuition fees to be paid. University regulations stipulate that the award of qualifications can be withheld if all outstanding debts to the university are not paid. Essential textbooks tend to be expensive and, due to demand, are often unavailable from libraries. Taking everything into account, being a student is an expensive business. Consequently, a majority of students run up considerable debts and have substantial overdrafts. Presently, the average medical undergraduate student debt is approximately £6,000 (Dangerfield, 2001) and the average dental student debt is £10,200 (British Dental Association, 2001). Although banks tend to be sympathetic they can sometimes refuse further credit, thereby causing concern. Financial hardship can weigh heavily on a student's conscience and financially induced stress can affect academic performance. Although most universities have hardship funds available, applications are strictly means-tested and the majority fail. Awareness of this discourages potential applicants. Loans and overdrafts eventually have to be repaid and qualifying with substantial debts is not the easiest start to a career.

Supporting graduate entrants to MDV education

There have always been mature students with non-clinical degrees who have subsequently sought to study the clinical disciplines. Special courses were set up for students who had not studied relevant GCSE A levels or whose degrees were not clinically related. With the government intent on increasing student numbers and widening access, numbers of graduate entrants will significantly increase. It is likely that these students will need even more support than undergraduates entering MDV education straight from school. Being a second degree, students will probably have to fund themselves entirely, including all tuition fees. Also, having a higher average age they may have other commitments such as a family to support. Becoming an undergraduate for the second time will almost certainly necessitate a reduction in income and create a greater need for an income-generating activity. Lifestyle may need to be changed. Children will need to be cared for whilst college activities are being undertaken and the strains of family life may cause problems in finding enough time for study.

Universities need to realize these problems and make the necessary allowances for supporting such students. For example, crèche facilities could be provided, and a more sympathetic response towards applications to hardship funds may be required. The circumstances of each student will need to be assessed individually and a learning plan or contract developed tailored to each individual's needs. This is where the tutor scheme could be of enormous benefit.

Accommodation

Living accommodation has to be arranged, and food and utility bills taken into account. Accommodation can have a profound effect on the ability to study. Most universities offer new undergraduates accommodation for at least their first year, usually in halls of residence. Some schools also offer bedsits, flats and shared houses for senior students. Student study bedrooms tend to be small and basically furnished, but at least they are a safe haven for someone until they have established themselves. They also tend to be relatively cheap. They should provide warmth, security, a reasonable degree of comfort, adequate bathroom facilities, adequate study facilities, be reasonably quiet for study and have communal areas.

Unfortunately, when large numbers of young people intent on enjoying their student lives to the full live together, the opportunity for peaceful study is often compromised! It is therefore important that student residences have wardens for arbitration when disputes arise.

Students often prefer to find their own accommodation in flats, or by collectively renting houses. Here they are not bound by the rules of university accommodation, only those of coexisting with themselves, neighbours and keeping the peace. Postgraduate students and graduate entrants to MDV education may have particular accommodation requirements that undergraduate facilities would not satisfy. For example, they may have families that require accommodation, or wish to share accommodation with a partner or spouse.

Poor accommodation, for whatever reason (discomfort, inadequate facilities, noise disturbance, disputes with flatmates), does have a profound effect upon psychological well-being and the ability to function well as a student.

Disability

Despite successfully completing the course and passing final examinations, deans of schools have to certify that successful students are fit for practice before the students can register with the relevant professional body (GMC, GDC, RVC). When applying for an undergraduate place, candidates must complete a health questionnaire that specifically asks about disabilities. If it can be shown that any existing disability is unlikely to affect a student's ability to perform their professional duties competently, that disability should not be used as a reason for the automatic rejection of the applicant. Despite enormous amounts of 'lip service' being paid to equalizing opportunities for students with disabilities, only limited resources have been made available. In law, universities are obliged to provide facilities for disabled students. There is some concern in MDV education about the potential for applications from students with disabilities considered incompatible with clinical practice. For example, it is presently inconceivable that a severely visually impaired person could practice as a surgeon. However, it is not inconceivable that such an individual would want to study medicine.

Students with mild disabilities (Ott, 1997) should not be barred from studying in MDV education if they can achieve the entrance requirements. For example, there have been many dyslexic students who have, with the support of their universities, become very successful practitioners.

Educational environment

The university is obliged to provide adequate support to enable each student to fulfil the educational requirements for their course of study. This would normally mean the provision of:

- a place for quiet study;
- library facilities;
- managed learning environment (MLE) – C&IT facilities (see Chapters 1 and 8);
- a meeting place;
- somewhere to eat (at reasonable cost);
- study rooms for lectures, seminars, tutorials that are adequately furnished and provided with relevant learning and teaching equipment;
- welfare (occupational health service, student counselling service, personal tutors).

Specific to medicine, dentistry and veterinary medicine are:

- clinical and laboratory facilities and equipment;
- access to patients, where relevant.

Professional behaviour

Aspiring students to the MDV professions are obliged to join strong professional cultures. They must comply with the mores of their chosen profession. Howley and Hartnett (1992) identified university pastoral powers over individuals as a form of coercion to impose compliance within the 'disciplines'. This contrasts with the process of teaching itself. They quote Foucault, who said that teaching gives 'access to the competing discourses that permit the care of the self, critique of official knowledge, and continuous elaboration of strategies of power'. This kind of argument emphasizes the importance of academic freedom, being mindful of the possible drawbacks of central prescribed institutional 'help' that can be seen as restrictive and controlling rather than liberating. The educational environment is constantly changing, as is the world of work and leisure outside. One line of logic from Barnett (2000) is that students should thus be drawn away from perceptions of permanence and be continually set problems in their education that convey the uncomfortable and uncertain territory they will have to adapt to in the future in order to be to be successful.

In MDV education 'acceptable' professional behaviour should always follow clear ethical guidelines intended to ensure that students and clinicians:

- show a duty of care to patients;
- respect issues of consent and confidentiality for patients, staff and students;

- are sensitive to issues of gender, race and disability;
- are prevented from taking unacceptable advantage of patients.

This represents a culture to which the student has to adapt (Bruffee, 1993). It can be difficult for some students from narrow, eurocentric class backgrounds to broaden their horizons, recognize their prejudices and realize the profession demands no unfair discrimination on any basis. Students with diverse cultural backgrounds may have difficulty making this adjustment, especially where they feel they are part of a minority group that needs to express itself and not be subjugated by what they may interpret as a white, male, middle-class dominated institution. For example, a most difficult adjustment could be for those students from cultures that limit the place and consideration of women in society. Male students will be expected to treat female patients with at least equal respect, and also respect and take advice from female academic and support staff. With a widening of student access and inclusivity and demands on the professions to become fairer and more equitable, misunderstandings are likely to increase rather than decrease with time.

Amelioration of some these issues could be achieved by improved communication as many may be misguided perceptions that need rational discussion. Clarification of what is expected of students, including the ability to accept positive criticism, is a vital function of the induction of students that should also be reinforced throughout the course. This should involve both staff and student participation and clear university-wide recognition and support. Situations can also arise where staff do not follow the espoused standards of their institutions and either exploit their position or treat others with prejudice. There should be no place for professional misconduct in the caring professions. Mechanisms must exist whereby anyone who perceives they are the victim of professional misconduct can appeal for help without fear of recrimination.

Ideally, an informal but defined approach to resolve conflicts between individuals, or between an individual and their university, should be available, eg, personal tutors or student counsellors. Where necessary, formal complaint procedures should be available that in no way reflect upon the character of any party until the complaint has been fully and impartially investigated. Unfortunately, students are generally reluctant to complain for fear of bias or even recrimination either from individual staff or on an institutional basis.

Collegiate support versus collegiate power

Students gain much support and motivation from enthusiastic academic and support staff (Race, 1998). In a recent workshop held in Cardiff, dental teachers were asked to rate what they thought characterized a good teacher. Enthusiasm, ability to communicate, knowledge of the discipline and interest were rated highly. Developing the right state of mind for learning is probably one of the most important issues for the individual student (Reinsmith, 1992).

Various curricular issues may affect student support directly. A competency-based curriculum can give each student a basis for confidence that they will be assessed with pre-defined criteria. The ethos of the curriculum should be to ensure that all will achieve core knowledge and skills to the appropriate standard so all should pass. In return, the obligations for the students will be articulated.

The value of interprofessional education in the development of professionals as team players has been recognized when it takes place in the real world, especially where allied healthcare professionals do work well together, such as in most interdisciplinary palliative care (Hall and Weaver, 2001). As yet there is little evidence for the role of interprofessional education as a source of support, although there is for some for the positive effects of peer support (Peat, Dalziel and Grant, 2001). Recognizing the value of other professions helps to place the professional goals of each student in perspective. A sustained mix of interprofessional development may place the students within reach of an appropriate environment for support, just at a time when this may not be available in their own profession.

'Curriculum stressors' are those items within the curriculum that a student may find difficult to cope with. On the medical side, role-modelling a patient and being physically examined (Braunack-Mayer, 2001), taking on the patient's disease sympathetically (Moss-Morris and Petrie, 2001) or breaking bad news without adequate training (Schildmann *et al*, 2001) have been found to be particularly stressful. Dental students may be worried by the prospect of hurting a patient or receiving critical remarks from a clinical supervisor. Veterinary students continually have to balance the needs of animal patients with the wishes of their owners. Care in dealing with identified sensitive issues within the curriculum can give support to students who will have to cope with these difficulties when they take up their profession after qualification.

MDV education involves producing team leaders who can take responsibility for their own learning, further development and support. What scope is there for developing self- and peer support? One of the most exciting projects to help with this will be the introduction of progress files as advocated in the *Dearing Report* (1997). A progress file will be made up of a transcript, personal development records and personal development planning. The whole purpose is to support students by making the fruits of their learning more explicit. The progress file transcript, kept by the university, will attempt to be far more detailed than current transcripts, thereby giving future employers far more detail about the achievements of the student. Personal development records indicate the importance given to personal reflection. Time and guidance from university sources should be made available for this private learning activity. Personal development planning is designed to encourage students to reflect upon and evaluate their own learning experiences and plan for their future development as part of the lifelong learning process.

All MDV education courses last a long time and the personal development planning part, in particular, may be useful for recording specialist options, extra-curricular activities and fieldwork that may prove relevant to a future career.

Personal development records have great potential for helping students manage curriculum stressors, as mentioned above. The problems of how essentially private reflection can be guided as a group activity and drawn into everyday life is exemplified in self-development methods (Progoff, 1992), but these have not yet been fully transferred into the higher education model.

Action learning sets (McGill and Beatty, 1995), which have been used successfully in the business and management world, may also prove useful in MDV education. These are small closed groups of individuals who meet on a regular basis to give each other time to express their current projects. Along the lines of the Kolb cycle of learning (see Chapters 4 and 11), colleagues never advise but prompt the presenter more towards reflection or action as appears appropriate.

Hub and spokes models

The image of the faceless university as a business trying to make ends meet, lecturers busy with research, and students trying somehow to gain an education has never been that stark in the smaller MDV Schools, where academic and administrative staff have worked together behind the scenes to support students. However, as Medical Schools expand they may have to consider concepts already used in the 'new universities' in an effort to maintain high retention levels. An example of a student 'hub and spokes' model is that of the 'student liaison officer'. The University of Central Lancashire has found this to be an excellent and cost-effective example of good practice in applied student support (Bratley, Francis and Wilson, 2001). They describe how three students took a year out after their second year to hold such faculty posts. Their aim was not to give advice, but to explain what options were available, thereby helping students in need to gain access to the correct information, enabling them to make their own decisions. Working unobtrusively in various ways, they helped the class representative system work better and relayed student feedback to academic staff.

Coventry University uses a 'hub and spokes' model whereby members of staff from the academic disciplines are brought into a central staff development unit for a year. It is this kind of secondment of relatively junior staff for involvement at the centre that could be so helpful in supporting administrative staff in the support of students. A percentage secondment from each department would make a start. The 'hub and spokes' would tend to democratize the process of student support in an MDV university and draw into the centre a healthy set of competing discourses.

Who should advise?

Most colleges of MDV education favour some form of tutor support for their students. Various tutor schemes prove very successful with the relatively small numbers of students involved in a dental clinical outpatients session, as described by Mullins, Wetherell and Robbé in Chapter 11. A centralized student advisory function may become more appropriate as MDV education numbers swell. Academics may find it useful to delegate module administration and time extensions to centrally placed or faculty administrative staff. A recent first conference on student advisory function in the United Kingdom reflected on the US model of developing academic advising as a separate profession that takes on the positive role of 'assisting students in the development of meaningful educational plans that are compatible with their life goals' (NACADA, 2001).

Tutors

A tutor is a member of staff responsible for the teaching and supervision of a certain number of students. There are many different types of tutor. For the support of students there are three different types – the academic tutor, the progress tutor and the personal tutor.

The academic tutor

An academic tutor is responsible, on a one-to-one basis, for supporting the learning of students. Sometimes this will also involve teaching. Not all faculties use the academic tutor system, simply relying on teachers to perform this role for their own specialities in the course. Alternatively students are not allocated tutors and are left to seek help from whoever they feel able to approach. A student may therefore have many different academic tutors (or none) in any year of study and throughout the course. Academic tutors are concerned only with the academic progress being made by their tutees in their specialist discipline, but should be able to report to student progress committees if necessary. Feedback to students could be in many different ways, for example, personal interview, written reports, comments on written work.

The progress tutor ('year tutor'; 'course tutor')

The progress tutor is concerned with monitoring student progress collectively. Their role is to collect, collate and analyse the summative and formative assessments for individual students and to report back to the university and to the student. They identify failing students and should attempt to institute remediation. They should also identify students making better than average progress. Often students are unaware of their formative assessments until some negative event brings critical reports to their attention. Again, not all MDV education schools use this system. The advantages of having progress tutors are:

- the early identification of weak or failing students;
- feedback for students;
- remediation when necessary;
- feedback for faculty and university;
- recognition and reward for students making good progress.

The personal tutor

Most universities have some form of personal tutor system whereby individual students are allocated to members of staff who are prepared to give help and advice when needed, ie, pastoral care. Training is necessary to prepare and motivate tutors to give enough support without being overbearing. The Quality Assurance Agency (QAA) recommends an effective personal tutor system for the identification of students who are failing in their chosen course for a variety of reasons other than academic ability. The personal tutor is meant to be the student's friend and advocate who will listen sympathetically in confidence and help and advise when necessary.

Traditionally the personal tutor receives progress reports for their tutees from the registry. They are supposed to meet with tutees several times throughout each academic year to discuss good or inadequate progress and to ascertain any mitigating circumstances if the student is failing. Ideally they act as a feedback mechanism for their tutees who are often unaware of the contents of formative reports. In practice this often results in personal tutors only interviewing students who are failing. Although personal tutors often do not honour their obligations to their tutees, the same applies to tutees not feeling inclined to seek out their personal tutors. There may be several reasons for this, not least of all lack of trust and worries about confidentiality on the part of the student. However, personal tutors also have a responsibility to inform their tutees of the mechanisms in place for supporting students, eg, the student counselling service.

One of the problems faced by personal tutors in the caring professions is the blurred distinction between tutoring and counselling. It is therefore essential that personal tutors receive adequate training for this role. The personal tutor can, at best, become a powerful ally for their tutees or, at least, a sympathetic listener and, as the old adage goes, a problem shared is a problem halved. It is important that tutees are informed of their progress on a regular basis and that there is a permanent, agreed record of the interview.

Feedback

Adequate support for all university students is essential if they are to be comfortable and, as a result, successful in their studies. How can universities ascertain that they are providing the necessary levels of support to achieve student comfort? An obvious method is to ask the students, either individually (eg, with questionnaires) or collectively by student representatives on teaching and learning committees. External examiners will often be able to judge the competency of students, thereby inferring a good working atmosphere. Mandatory reviews of academic institutions by government bodies take student feedback into consideration when preparing their recommendations. MDV Schools are regularly 'visited' by the regulatory bodies (GMC, GDC, RVC) to ensure that professional standards are being maintained and these visitations take into account comments from student representatives.

Self-help

Students will naturally seek help from other students, mainly from their peers, but also from more experienced students within their faculty. Simply talking to other students allows reflection on one's own progress and level of achievement. Students find this less threatening and much more comfortable than a formal approach to academic staff. This emphasizes the importance of facilitating ways in which students can interact with each other.

Supporting postgraduate students

Postgraduate or research students have progressed to a higher level of education – that of independent learning and being able to contribute to the general body of knowledge in their chosen field of study. Traditionally, postgraduate students carried out a research project of their own choosing, assisted by a supervisor, which resulted in a postgraduate qualification, together with a published thesis (Diploma, Masters degree, Doctorate). Presently there are an increasing number of taught postgraduate courses that lead to a registerable qualification as part of a professional career pathway but there is usually an associated research thesis that contributes towards the final assessment.

Postgraduate students tend to work alone and are often more isolated than undergraduates. They tend to lack a sense of belonging and often find collective interaction with fellow students difficult, especially if they did not gain their first degree at their chosen research university. It is therefore important for postgraduate students to have some means of interacting with other students within their faculty or through a postgraduate society. Distance learning courses are also growing in popularity but here the sense of isolation can be even more marked. Support for distance learning students can be problematical but the university should make an effort to provide support mechanisms, should the distance learners wish to take advantage of them. Of paramount importance for the research postgraduate student is the correct choice of institution and supervisor where they intend to pursue their studies.

Responsibilities of research students

Postgraduate students would normally be expected to define their chosen area of research, be knowledgeable in the subject chosen (literature review) and produce a detailed framework and timetable for the proposed research (Cryer, 2000). They should choose the topics they wish to discuss with their supervisor in timetabled meetings and be prepared to accept feedback and guidance. Written work should be submitted for appraisal punctually, as agreed in their learning contract.

Responsibilities of supervisors

Postgraduate students expect their supervisors to be available when needed, read their submitted work both carefully and punctually, give constructive (rather than destructive) feedback and have a good knowledge of their research area. Local knowledge on availability of patients or research materials and realistic timescales for projects are particularly valuable resources for a new postgraduate in the medical field. They should show interest in the student's area of research and help with the provision of information (Phillips and Pugh, 2000). They also expect help towards finding post-research employment. Students dislike supervisors who are constantly adding to their workload irrelevant ideas outside the chosen research field.

It is now generally accepted that research supervisors need training and staff development. Supervisors would normally be expected to have knowledge of the research subject area and theoretical approach to be applied. They should regularly and formally meet with their students, help in the planning of the research project (involving other experts, if necessary) and advise on lectures or courses that may aid their student's research. They should read and critically appraise written work as it is produced, monitor their student's progress and give valid feedback. Supervisors should maintain a record of progress for each student and regularly report on progress to the higher degrees committee.

Responsibilities of the university

Postgraduate students are largely responsible for their own integration into the educational institution. However, the university is obliged to provide support. Every postgraduate student should have access to office accommodation, library and IT facilities. Ideally there should also be communal facilities for refreshment breaks and the opportunity to meet informally with staff and other students. Laboratory and workshop facilities should also be provided, where appropriate.

Student counselling service

All students in higher education should have access to a professional counselling service where they can seek help and advice with absolute confidentiality.

Counselling is a specific skill that, ideally, should only be undertaken by trained counsellors. Poor counselling can lead to a course of action that results in adverse rather than beneficial outcomes. Students with personal problems often feel unable to discuss them with academic staff or personal tutors as they feel that there may be a lack of confidentiality. Alternatively, their problems may be of such a sensitive nature that they would not like to discuss them with someone they know as a teacher, a friend or even a parent. For example, drugs, alcohol, personal relationships and debt. They need to discuss their problems with someone impartial who will not necessarily tell them what they should do, but rather facilitate access to all necessary information so that informed decisions can be made as to future actions.

Sometimes students find the initial approach to professional counselling difficult. Students may be unaware that a counselling service is available, despite being given details (eg, in student handbooks) at their induction. Occasionally teaching staff may suggest that a student should visit the counselling service, especially when the student makes the initial approach, if they feel the scope of the problem is outside their remit as a teacher or personal tutor. The emphasis for good communication is therefore placed on the university. Not only should information be readily available for students but also staff, and especially personal tutors, should be made aware of the counselling service. They can (and should) then inform their tutees of its availability and scope.

Conclusion

The range and depth of student support in MDV education should be increased and improved following political moves to widen access and greatly increase the numbers of qualified practitioners. Support needs to be provided centrally at the institutional level, and also at faculty, departmental, and individual levels. The utilization of professional support staff at administrative level could help MDV universities become more efficient in supporting students and in dealing with student problems as and when they arise.

Opportunities for the training of support staff are presently available. Some examples are the Staff and Educational Development Association (SEDA) postgraduate certificate, National Vocational Qualifications (NVQs) in Counselling Skills and the Training and Accreditation Programme for Postgraduate Supervisors (TAPPS).

Provision of a comprehensive professional support service is a desirable aim, but the uptake of this service could be problematical. The recruitment of additional liaison staff from experienced students and newly qualified staff could be an innovative way in helping students access the support they need.

References

Barnett, R (2000) *Realizing the University in an age of Supercomplexity*, Society for Research in Higher Education and Open University Press, Buckingham

Bratley, S, Francis, P and Wilson, L (2001) Bridging the Gap, *Proceedings of the First Annual Conference on Academic Advising*, Luton University

Braunack-Mayer, A (2001) Should medical students act as surrogate patients for each other?, *Medical Education*, **35**, pp 681–86

British Dental Association (BDA) Research Unit (2001) *Student Debt Survey*, London

Bruffee, K (1993) *Collaborative Learning: Higher Education, interdependence, and the authority of knowledge*, The Johns Hopkins University Press, Baltimore and London

Cryer, P (2000) *The Research Student's Guide to Success*, 2nd edn, Open University Press, Buckingham

Dangerfield, P (2001) Medical student debt in the United Kingdom, *Medical Education*, **35**, pp 619–21

Dearing, R (1997) *Report of the National Committee of Inquiry into Higher Education*, Chapter 9, p 20, NCIHE Publications, London

Duguid, R (1989) Applications and admissions to UK dental schools through UCCA: 1968–1987, *British Dental Journal*, **167**, pp 337–400

Hall, P and Weaver, L (2001) Interdisciplinary education and teamwork: a long and winding road, *Medical Education*, **35**, pp 867–75

Howley, A and Hartnett, R (1992) Pastoral Power and the Contemporary University: A Foucauldian Analysis, *Educational Theory*, **42,** pp 1–13

McGill, I and Beaty, L (1995*) Action Learning: A guide for professional, management and educational development*, 2nd edn, Kogan Page, London

Moss-Morris, R and Petrie, K (2001) Redefining medical students' disease to reduce morbidity, *Medical Education*, **35,** pp 724–28

NACADA (The National Academic Advising Association) (2001) *Professional Resources* [Online] http://www.nacada.ksu.edu/Profres/resources2.html.

Ott, P (1997) *How to Detect and Manage Dyslexia: a reference and resource manual*, Heinemann, London

Peat, M, Dalziel, J and Grant, A (2001) Enhancing the First Year Student Experience by Facilitating the Development of Peer Networks through a One-day Workshop, *Higher Education Research and Development*, **20,** pp 199–215

Phillips, E and Pugh, D (2000) *How to Get a PhD*, 3rd edn, Open University Press, Buckingham

Progoff, I (1992) *At a Journal Workshop*, Putnam, New York

Race, P (1998) Teaching: creating a thirst for learning?, in *Motivating Students*, ed S Brown, S Armstrong and G Thompson, pp 47–57, Kogan Page, London

Reinsmith, W (1992) *Archetypal Forms in Teaching: A Continuum*, Greenwood Press, Westport, Connecticut

Schildmann, J *et al* (2001) Evaluation of a 'breaking bad news' course at the Charité, Berlin, *Medical Education*, **35,** pp 806–07

Sjostrom, O (1995) Number of applicants and examination frequency at the dental schools in Sweden 1968–1992, *Swedish Dental Journal*, **19**, pp 219–24

University of Wales College of Medicine (UWCM) (2001) UWCM launches Compact Scheme to Widen Access, *The Bulletin:* the newsletter for staff and associates of UWCM, pp 7–8, UWCM, Cardiff

10

Learning environments – a teacher's strategy

Ronald Brown and John Sweet

Introduction

Throughout MDV education, new curricula are being developed that favour a learning and teaching strategy concerned with good communication, generic skills training, core competences, student-chosen specialist options and group study skills for lifelong learning. For this to happen, traditional subject courses have to be shortened, particularly in the basic sciences and in those that entail memorizing facts or carrying out procedures that are not core or central to professional education. Some course leaders, suddenly come up against a situation where they are given less time in which to 'cover' their syllabus. However, the ability of students to 'uncover' information and understanding in the subject for themselves may be far more important in their professional lives (Wilby, 2001).

Using the working example of dental undergraduate technology as a model, this chapter attempts to show how the teacher can become an agent for change, and use the situation to draw on educational experience and evidence to provide a learning environment in a condensed but more focussed course. The specific detailed examples of the components of a dental technology course are located in text boxes so that the chapter can be read from a general MDV context by reading the main text and skimming the specific subject content in the boxes.

Dental undergraduate education in technology

Most undergraduate regulatory bodies are currently recommending that students should experience sufficient exposure to technical training to be able to prescribe a full range of crowns, bridges and dentures (GDC, 1997). Whether students should ever need to construct a set of complete dentures in the future is contentious. The number of edentulous patients is declining in many countries: from 30 per cent in 1968 to around 13 per cent in 2001 in the United Kingdom (Royal Society of Edinburgh, 2001). If the demand for the provision of complete dentures becomes low, Bertolami (2001) argues that postgraduate dental specialists should carry them out. An alternative would be to delegate this to specially trained clinical technicians. Even if the dental student performs the routine clinical aspects of constructing dentures, it is doubtful that they would ever have to carry out the technical aspects and so would not need to pursue the technical methodology, in any great depth. The 'core' focus in the prosthetic field for dental undergraduate education must therefore be history and examination, diagnosis and clinical stages of denture construction, rather than technical processes.

On the technical side, the challenge is to develop in the student sufficient appreciation of theoretical and practical aspects of technical work so that they are able to make a detailed prescription for the technician to construct a prosthesis. Following this, the student should be able to identify prostheses that have been made to that specification but more importantly, be able to recognize when and in what way they have been made in an unsatisfactory manner. It is also essential that they can understand sufficient theory and know enough about the practicalities of the construction of prostheses. They would then be able to appraise critically the work produced by the technician, and be able to make recommendations for modification where necessary. This philosophy is very different from some current undergraduate dental courses that include detailed technical training. More progressive dental courses release time for clinical and academic work, expecting the technical experience to be completed in a shorter time. The ability and willingness to help the student command a more appropriate focussed view on technical work is a particular challenge to the lecturer or instructor in dental technology.

Just as higher education institutions will have a strategy for learning and teaching, so will the individual teacher have a strategy for their own learning and teaching. As Biggs (1999) indicates, teachers may take on the institutional mandate but have to work out their own solutions. The need for reciprocity is identified when he later goes on to say, 'The individual teacher improves through reflecting on current practice through the lenses of an operating theory; so should the institution'

(Biggs, 2001). The strategy for teachers is therefore both to follow the institutional learning and teaching strategy and reflect on their current practice and on current educational recommendations and evidence to develop a flexible philosophy of teaching that will empower their students' learning. We set out our own philosophy of teaching in the anagram EDUCATION in Table 10.1 below.

Table 10.1 Teaching philosophy – EDUCATION

Features to be encouraged	Possible learning activities
Enjoyment	educational games example crossword puzzles
Dedication	assignments and self-directed learning
Understanding	debates
Collaboration	collaborative learning and PBL
Assessment	formative and summative assessment
Thought-provoking	plenary session to follow buzz groups
Innovation	buzz groups, reverse pyramiding
Observation	self-, peer and group criticism
Never-ending	professionalism and lifelong learning

EDUCATION should be **E** as enjoyable as possible. Creating a non-threatening and supportive educational environment for the students can enhance enjoyment experienced, with time protected for critical learning individual and group activities, which can include games (for example, discipline-based crossword puzzles). Learning needs **D** dedication. This can be enhanced by allocating some work that, as well as being assessed, will encourage self-directed learning, aiming to draw the student towards a state of 'learning for the love of it'. It is not just knowledge but **U** understanding that is important. Debates, in which differing views are presented and yet where a consensus judgement is secured, can help students appreciate others' views and further understanding. **C** is for collaboration that can be achieved by appropriate facilitation of learning in small groups, where individuals rely on one another to gain valuable learning experience. Assessment **A** should be carried out both during learning as an aid to learning for formative feedback, and as a summative exercise to accredit achievement of learning. Teaching should be **T** for thought-provoking. One approach to stimulating thinking is the gathering of small groups into a plenary session, to compare and contrast their different views. Each educational situation is unique and invites the teacher to exploit the educational opportunities with **I** innovation. Observation **O** and reflection are key learning elements. Students and staff should be open to self- and peer appraisal, and wherever possible group appraisal. Never-ending **N** is the final strand of educational philosophy, stressing the need for continuing professional education of teachers and the goals of enthusing students for lifelong learning.

Once the model for educational development has been drawn up, priority can be given to changing or creating specific course elements. It then remains a matter of putting ideas into action.

Teaching strategy

In MDV education, the teaching focus must ultimately be on patient need and possibly on the other stakeholders in a patient's welfare and this must be remembered when designing or improving a course. Teachers should follow the agreed professional guidelines and learning and teaching strategies of the institution where they work. In addition, teachers will use their own teaching philosophy when making decisions on the content of a course and the methods used to facilitate and appraise learning. In order to draw out clearly the general issues that could apply to any MDV topic, the strategy used to design the dental technology course will be explained in terms of concept and evidence. The decision to apply a concept to the course is described in open text and flagged with heading 'Concept'. The source of the andragogical (adult educational) evidence that is applied here is also described in open text and flagged with the heading 'Evidence'. Detail on how this evidence may be incorporated into or applied to the dental technology course is shown in the text boxes.

Concept 1 – The overall picture

Students should be given an opportunity to briefly experience an overview of the course, to understand what it entails, what is expected of them during the learning activities, and in general, what the learning outcomes are and how they will be measured.

Evidence 1

Ausubel (1978), campaigned for meaningful learning as a reaction against 'rote memorizing' commonly used at that time. He showed that organization of knowledge was important for meaningful learning and that a 'background knowledge' of concepts and principles was essential for problem-solving. He recommended the use of advance organizers; a presentation of the entire content in its final form, to be used at the very start of a course. Anchoring of specific detail can then follow in ways that permit essential links between the parts (see also Curzon, 2000).

1 Dental technology example – course outline

As an introduction to the making of dentures, the students are given access to videos and slides, which show both the clinical and technical stages involved. These techniques are also illustrated in the handbook provided for student use, which contains suitable places for students to add queries at the start of their studies and later as a workbook, a place for more reflective comments.

Concept 2 – Competency statements and specific learning objectives and learning outcomes

Clear statements that set out core competency requirements for a new graduate, and more detailed learning outcomes for specific courses, can help the student to keep a focus on learning appropriate skills, and help reduce course overload.

Evidence 2

Kirschner *et al* (1997) set out the case for a study environment in higher education where there is a development of academic and professional competence. They formulate competence to mean that knowledge and skills have been acquired to a sufficient minimum standard. Biggs (1999) emphasizes the importance of a focus on 'how well' students know, as much as 'what' they know. Specifying learning objectives in advance of their attainment does not preclude other desirable but unforeseen outcomes. Prosser and Trigwell (1998) also argue for the quality of learning outcomes, which they equate with 'ways of understanding'. Students should be able to see relations between elements of their understanding, and that these relationships can be applied in new ways in novel situations. Students need to be drawn into the educational process so that they can understand how they can use the directives to their greatest advantage.

2 Examples of competency statements and objectives for dental technology

Competency statements adapted from AADS (1999):

Restore partial or complete edentulous patients with uncomplicated fixed or removable prostheses.
Communicate case design with laboratory technicians and evaluate the resultant prosthesis.

Learning objectives:
To be able to describe the engineering principles related to constructing a cast cobalt/chrome partial denture with special reference to fulcrums, levers and the limitations of metals to be used.
To be able to survey and design acrylic and metal partial dentures and provide a coherent prescription for a dental technician either in writing or verbally.

The student workbook contains all the competency statements and specific learning objectives with room for reflections and annotations. Reference is made to them as a class activity.

Concept 3 – How to learn something practical

Students with a range of ability and approach can be supported to reach adequate levels of psychomotor skills by applying modern conceptions and evidence from research. Enlightened approaches may prevent less able students from an early sense of failure to perform, compared with their more successful peers.

Evidence 3

Dick and Carey (1990) provide some insight into learning psychomotor skills, which, in contrast to cognitive learning, they see as a linear progression of initial plans of interest, through various actions to an evaluation or feedback based on the outcomes of actions. They recommend the use of job-aids – which the learner can refer to in order to gain just the right amount of information needed for that procedure, and so prevent student information overload. Curzon (2000) recommends that psychomotor skills lessons should have a structure of approximately 25 per cent demonstration, 15 per cent verbal explanation and 60 per cent guided practice. The content of courses that develop skills must be 'authentic', as Feil, Reed and Hart (1990) have shown that skills are very context-specific. For instance, skills developed in the laboratory where dentures are made, will not be transferred to the situation of restoring a decayed tooth in the dental clinic.

Considerable insight into the acquisition of psychomotor skills is given by Mayberry *et al* (1993) in their model of motor skill learning. The model is centred on the need for the student to visualize and have an accurate representation of the desired outcome. There is a case here to leave the 'common sense' practice and start the teaching process from the final outcome, working backwards through the sequence of actions and processes to the beginning and only then defining the initial conditions required for success. In addition to the outcome, there needs to be a visualization of the procedure. This is clearly where a demonstration, going through the stages from start to finish, is invaluable. Dick and Carey's (1990) model focusses on correctness and would discard error. Mayberry *et al* (1993) set knowledge of results, the comparison between actual and desired outcomes, as critical in the learning process.

Certainly, in a laboratory or simulated clinical situation, error can be celebrated as useful information that can be shared and evaluated with others. A common fault, to which others can be alerted, may prevent them from making this error themselves. The Mayberry *et al* (1993) model emphasizes the importance of process as well as outcome; the means to the end must be evaluated and justified.

3 Order of teaching

To allow the students to assimilate course requirements, they are shown an overview of all the various stages of denture construction and given explanations for the different stages. This acts as a template for visual and mental representation of the desired outcome, which they can compare to their actual outcomes. This should enhance the students' performance. Students can then be given practical demonstrations, which will allow them to assess the lecturers' performance and discuss whether the desired criteria have been met. If the students fail to recognize any flaw either deliberate or otherwise it is the demonstrator's obligation to point out these faults.

These laboratory courses use manikins (phantom heads) to simulate the patient in the clinical situation, as well as using students themselves as models to take impressions. The students then perform the exercise under close supervision.

Concept 4 – Structured group learning

Group objective structured clinical examination, normally an assessment method, can be adapted to be a method of group learning to evaluate common errors and improve knowledge of results. The work stations and objects can also provide a focus for brainstorming with the students integrating their ideas in order to provide an action plan for those demonstrating errors.

Evidence 4

Harden and Gleeson (1979) were the first to describe the objective structured clinical examination (OSCE), a standardized test for individual students based on their performance at a series of clinical stations. This was developed as a group activity by Biran (1991) and called Group OSCE (GOSCE) and used later by Elliot *et al* (1994). These authors stress the advantage that this group process permits feedback to be given more easily than the time-consuming procedure for individuals. If the assessment and clinical aspects are abandoned, the procedure can be turned into a teaching method in practically any subject to provide an opportunity for a group learning.

4 Group objective structured laboratory learning (GOSLL)

The student group is presented with objects on a laboratory bench such as dental models and dentures at various stages of completion. In addition to exemplars, some objects demonstrate constructional faults. The challenge is for the group to be able to order the items correctly to show the chain of events in denture construction. In addition, they must identify the severity of technical faults and means to rectify these where possible. The collection of objects with a range of errors shows the value of all products of the students' activity for learning, whatever the results. A clearer vision of desired outcome and a knowledge of results help the students to evaluate the technician's work.

Concept 5 – Collaborative and self-directed learning

Collaborative learning occurs when all the members of a group have an opportunity to contribute and take responsibility for each other's learning. Self-directed learning occurs when individuals take responsibility for their own learning. Both processes are learner- as opposed to teacher-based and reflect the situation that will exist when the new graduate is practising, learning from experience and many other resources, both as an individual and as part of a healthcare team.

Evidence 5

Caffarella (1993) sees many positive effects of self-directed learning and the sense of autonomy it creates: students show independence and can make decisions. He also claims that in the process, students are able to reach a further depth of character; be able to articulate clearly the range of learning activities that they can undertake and develop a strong sense of personal values and beliefs. A further claim is coupled with two aspects of collaborative learning, namely, interdependence and interconnectedness.

Bruffee (1994) emphasizes that positive interdependence is a learned craft where students learn whilst constructing knowledge, to depend upon one another, rather than depending exclusively on the authority of the teacher. Whilst group activities are widely held as peripheral events and social activities, in most organizations the new concept here is to place the collaborative effort within the classroom (the learning environment), which classically has been the centre for individual competitive activity. Johnson and Johnson (1999) from their research in schools, find that optimal learning can take place in an environment of positive interdependence, but this does not exclude the possibility of using competition between small groups to enhance motivation.

Boyer (1989) stressed the importance of what he called 'connectedness'. His was a vision of how education should, through good communication, draw individuals together to share information and pursue collaborative problem-solving. Far from leaving the students to their own devices, except possibly with the help of some computer package, he stipulated that, in the end, teachers who serve as models and mentors establish connectedness. In essence, the teacher needs to create materials and an environment where individual students can negotiate their role in the collaborative effort. This may involve the selection of a topic for self-directed learning that they will later report on to the whole group. The focus is kept on the learners by asking them to present their findings, with the role of the facilitator being to ensure that the objectives of the activity are met to an adequate level.

5 Sharing information about the periodontal/prosthetic interface jigsaw

This work is carried out in a small group with roles for the membership, which includes chairperson, scribe and timekeeper (teaching materials are given in writing):

- A good published review article on the periodontal/prosthetic interface is divided into six sections so that, for a group of 12 students, one pair of students will be allocated each section.
- The relevant sections are given out to the pairs of students for self-study and research, with a requirement that a short presentation will be necessary at a future group meeting.
- At the meeting, the learning objectives are agreed and pairs of students are given 15 minutes to prepare a joint presentation.
- Each pair presents a section on the paper for three or four minutes with a few minutes for questions (30 minutes in all).
- There is discussion and feedback to confirm that the learning objectives have been met.

Concept 6 – Changing group dynamics to improve learning – reverse pyramiding

Undertaking practical tasks can appear to be a tremendous hurdle for some students. A purposeful structured group activity can often help mobilize group strengths that can support and draw individuals along. A structured group approach can provide a sensitive response to the 'natural' inclination to prefer the anonymity of larger groups at some points in the learning process. At other times, learning may be served better by a very small group, which permits cohesiveness and support to achieve a common purpose.

Evidence 6

Jacques (2000) describes how snowballs or pyramid groups can be built up, starting with individual students writing down their ideas on paper. At a second stage, they can share their ideas in pairs. As the groups enlarge, they can also engage in increasingly complex tasks to avoid repetition. The pairs can then be doubled into fours and finally eights, which can then report back to a plenary session. We use the reverse logic with a reverse pyramiding technique. Colleagues provide support and positive criticism in small groups, which are systematically halved, until the student is working competently alone.

6 Pyramiding and reverse pyramiding

The class is split up into small groups of four and each student is provided with a different plaster model showing teeth with spaces for a partial denture. This allows the students to help each other to produce an outline denture design. After a period of discussion, the group is cut by 50 per cent. The student pairs continue a joint discussion until the individual students feel confident enough to carry out a detailed denture design drawing on their own. To complete the learning loop, the students can return to their original groups of four to assess their own and each other's designs.

Concept 7 – Self- and peer assessment

MDVE students will become clinical practitioners who have to make decisions for themselves based on a self-assessment. For instance, a decision to continue treatment or to refer could be of critical importance to a patient. However, some care is carried out more in teams and it is in this situation that it is essential to give and accept constructive criticism. Carefully organized peer assessment of student work may provide practice in this regard.

Evidence 7

Brown, Bull and Pendlebury (1997) make the point that self- and peer assessment are not methods of assessment but sources of assessment in which a number of methods or instruments may be used. Boud (1995) suggests that self-assessment be carried out in two parts: firstly to set the criteria for assessment, and secondly to perform the assessment based on the criteria. Boud thinks that peer assessment should be used to inform but advises against students grading each other. As Brew (1999) states, peer assessment is very different from self-assessment, and involves further processes and potential hazards. Clearly, students may dislike making judgements about their colleagues and may not have developed sufficient skills to either perform an assessment or give appropriate feedback. Boud (1995) says that feedback should be useful but is strongly against phoney or contrived praise that is patronizing and controlling. Rather, in a memorable turn of phrase, he says that peer assessment should 'affirm the worth of the person and give support whilst offering reactions to the object of attention'.

7 Self- and peer assessed laboratory exercises

- The students as a group generate the criteria for successful completion of the exercise, based on the learning objectives, demonstrations, and tutor support given during the session. The end product to be assessed is usually a dental model with a design or object such as a crown or denture at some stage of construction fitting on to it.
- The criteria are prioritized.
- The criteria are weighted if necessary and a marking scheme devised.
- Students assess their own laboratory exercise based on the weighted marking scheme.
- A pair of students evaluate each other's laboratory work based on the agreed criteria, and make appropriate comments to their peer, who may adjust their self-assessed mark based on this further peer information.

Concept 8 – Learning from experience

Students often find it hard to see links between one subject and another. Integration of subjects and practical application can help.

Evidence 8

Kolb (1984) states that learning from experience is essential for individual and organizational effectiveness. Students need to learn an appropriate response to their patients needs. Kolb says all learning is based on the process of inhibition of incorrect responses. Whilst this particular quote may be an overstatement, input to appreciate the patient's position (such as wearing an appliance) is of great value in managing their needs. Further insight into learning from experience comes from Heron (1996) who distinguishes factual, practical, intuitive grasp of patterns and experiential knowing the presence of a person or thing.

8 Clinical/laboratory interface

This is a structured exercise to allow the students to design, construct and wear various denture-like appliances. There is an opportunity here to practice working with clinical and laboratory dental materials, to experience the overall sensation of wearing a prosthesis and to study the effects on the periodontal tissues. The class is divided into three groups to construct an appliance:

- designed to cover the gums but relieved so not to press on them;
- designed to cover and rest on the gums;
- designed to have minimal contact with teeth and gums.

Each student will have an oral examination by their peers before and after the appliance is inserted. Students will be instructed in hygiene techniques for cleaning the appliance. They will then wear the appliance for a two-week period. After this period, the students will then examine each other for inflammation of the gingival tissue, for levels of plaque accumulation and soft or hard tissue damage. They will reflect on the experience of wearing the appliance, write these in their workbooks and share their experiences in a group discussion.

Concept 9 – Student assessment of teaching

Whilst learners must take responsibility for their own learning, there are times when teaching support to facilitate learning may be critical. The kind of impact teaching has on the student experience can vary and may not be obvious to the lecturer.

Evidence 9

There was a surge of interest in student feedback in the 1980s and 1990s with a centrally funded student feedback system project centred at Loughborough (King, 2000). They documented a range of methods from informal channels and staff/student committees to questionnaires, including open and closed questions and free comments. King also points out that it is essential that academic staff voluntarily reflect on their teaching and develop what they do. He also sees the completion of a feedback loop from the lecturers' response to the students' evaluation as a crucial exercise. He also notes that care should be taken that students' reactions to unpopular topics are not taken as personal responses to a teacher's ability.

9 Joint formal and informal assessment

Modules of the dental technology course are evaluated by students with a questionnaire filled in at a debriefing last session. With reference to the original learning objectives for the module, questions are asked of:

- **Self**: What and how well did I learn in this module and what did I achieve?
- **Group**: How well did the group as a whole learn and what did it achieve?
- **Peers**: How did the colleagues I worked with learn and what did they achieve?
- **Tutor**: How well did the tutor facilitate learning?
- **Module topic**: Did the examples chosen to illustrate the topic appear well-chosen? Would the module have been better integrated elsewhere in the course?

Once completed, students and tutors can informally discuss their findings.

Conclusion

This chapter aimed to show that even if a topic has been demoted in terms of time allocation, a fresh emphasis on teaching strategy can help a focussed shortened course become a useful resource for the student. It also aimed to show that the andragogical and other educational literature can provide evidence for actions to take to improve learning. There still remains the challenge and risks of attempting something new with our students in our particular situation and the importance of gaining feedback from them on the initiatives taken.

References

AADS 1998–1999 Annual Proceedings, *Journal of Dental Education*, **63** (7), pp 565–67

AADS (1999) *Exhibit 6 – Competencies for the New Dentist*

Ausubel, D (1978) *Educational Psychology – a Cognitive View*, Holt, Rinehart and Winston, New York

Bertolami, C N (2001) Rationalizing the Dental Curriculum in Light of Current Disease Prevalence and Patient Demand for Treatment: Form vc Content, *Journal of Dental Education*, **65** (8), pp 725–35

Biggs, J (1999) *Teaching for quality learning at university: What the student does*, SRHE and OUP, Buckingham

Biggs, J (2001) On What to Teach: Clarifying Objectives, *University of Edinburgh* [Online] www.ltsn.ac.uk/news/News_items/OnConstructiveAlignment_John%20Biggs.rtf

Biran, L A (1991) Self-assessment and learning through GOSCE (group objective structured clinical examination), *Medical Education*, **25** (6), pp 475–79

Boud, D (1995) *Enhancing Learning through Self Assessment*, reprint 1997, ed Kogan Page, London

Boyer, E L (1989) Connectedness Through Liberal Education, in *Curriculum Planning: A New Approach*, ed G Hass, F Parkay, 6th edn, pp 525–31, Allyn and Bacon, Boston

Brew, A (1999) Towards Autonomous Assessment: Using Self-Assessment and Peer Assessment, in *Assessment Matters in Higher Education: Choosing and Using Diverse Approaches*, eds S Brown, A Glaser, pp 159–71, SRHE, London

Brown, G, Bull, J, Pendlebury, M (1997) *Assessing Student Learning in Higher Education*, 1st edn, Routledge, London

Bruffee, K A (1993) *Collaborative Learning: Higher Education, Interdependence, and the Authority of Knowledge*, 1995 edn, The John Hopkins University Press, Baltimore and London

Caffarella, R S (1993) Self-Directed Learning, in *New Directions for Adult and Continuing Education*, edn v, **57**, pp 25–35, Jossey-Bass, San Francisco

Curzon, B L (2000) *Teaching in Further Education*, 5th edn, Pippin Publishing Corporation, London

Dick, W and Carey, L (1990) *The Systematic Design of Instruction*, 3rd edn, Harper Collins

Elliot, D L, Fields, S A, Keenen, T L *et al* (1994) Use of a Group Objective Structured Examination with First-year Medical Students, *Academic Medicine*, **69**, pp 990–92

Feil, P, Reed, T and Hart, J K (1990) The transfer effect of lead up activities, *Journal of Dental Education*, **54** (10), pp 609–11

GDC (1997) *The First Five Years: The Undergraduate Dental Curriculum*, London

Harden, R M, Gleeson, F A (1979) Assessment of Clinical Competence Using Objective Structured Clinical Examination, *Medical Education*, **13**, pp 41–54

Heron, J (1996) *Co-operative Inquiry: Research into the human condition*, Sage, London

Jacques, D (2000) *Learning in Groups: A handbook for improving group work*, Kogan Page, London

Johnson, D W and Johnson, R T (1999) *Learning Together and Alone*, 5th edn, Allyn and Bacon, Boston

King, M (2000) *Student Feedback Systems: Approach to Feedback* [Online] http://www.lboro.ac.uk/service/sd/sfs/loughbor.htm

Kirschner, P, Van Vilsteren, P, Hummel, H *et al* (1997) The Design of a Study Environment for Acquiring Academic and Professional Competence, *Studies in Higher Education*, **22**, pp 151–71

Kolb, D A (1984) *Experiential learning experience as the source of learning and development*, Prentice-Hall, Englewood Cliffs

Mayberry, W E *et al* (1993) *An Introduction to Problem-Based Learning*, University Missouri-Kansas

Prosser, M and Trigwell, K (1998) *Understanding Learning and Teaching: The Experience in Higher Education*, Open University Press, Buckingham

Royal Society of Edinburgh (2001) *Dental Health in the Older Adult: A Neglected Issue* [Online] http://www.ma.hw.ac.uk/RSE/meetingsetc/conf2001/oralhealthabst.htm copy

Wilby, P (2001) 'It is not what you cover but what you uncover that is important', quotation at MSc Module in Continuing Professional Development University of Wales College of Medicine

11

Learning in the clinical environment

Gerry Mullins, John Wetherell and Iain Robbé

Introduction

The clinic is the learning environment to which all our students aspire. It is the arena in which our early educational preparation is centred to provide sufficient skills, knowledge and professionalism to enable our fledgling dentists to treat patients. Although, in this chapter, we make frequent reference to dental education, the same principles apply to medicine and veterinary science. The outcomes for our professions are the same in that our goal as educators is to prepare competent, confident and knowledgeable practitioners and lifelong learners.

In the past, clinical learning was reserved for the later years of medical, dental and veterinary (MDV) courses. It was considered necessary to have all the basic sciences and theoretical concepts in place before students could see patients. However, in the early 1990s we conducted a survey of our students throughout all years of the 'old'/conventional curriculum. From students in the earlier, pre-clinical years of the course, we received many negative comments relating to heavy contact hours, redundant material and a perceived lack of relevance of theory to practice. Students arrived at the clinic with a vast theoretical knowledge from their subject-centred, pre-clinical education, to be faced with the contrast of problem-oriented, practical experience (Townsend *et al*, 1997). Other reasons for a change in the curriculum were also evident at this time:

- an explosion of knowledge in the biodental and biomedical sciences generating new philosophies and controversies in patient care;

- dramatic changes in the health of the Australian population, with marked reductions in dental caries in younger individuals and an increasing proportion of middle-aged/elderly dentate and medically compromised patients;
- significant technological advances, including new restorative and implant materials that have broadened the available range of treatment options;
- major advances in the field of teaching methodology, including the availability of computer-assisted learning (CAL) and multimedia technology.

Similar pressures for change have been seen in medical and veterinary courses. For example, the General Medical Council (GMC, 1993), the UK statutory body for medical undergraduate education, has required major changes to the medical curriculum in order to promote the exploration of knowledge, learning by curiosity, critical evaluation of evidence and a capacity for self-education, amongst other things. In response to the recommendations of the GMC, Medical Schools throughout the United Kingdom have changed their curricula, and the University of Wales College of Medicine (UWCM) (1994) replaced the traditional curriculum with the integrated curriculum, which has better links between scientists and clinicians, more learner-centred and problem-orientated teaching, and an emphasis on helping students to acquire learning skills as well as medical knowledge.

In response to developments in dentistry, a new five-year, PBL-based curriculum was introduced at Adelaide Dental School. It commenced with first year in 1993, and was progressively introduced, one year at a time, until 1997, so that the methods and processes described here are well established, and documented in Mullins *et al* (2001a).

Because of these basic philosophical and educational changes in the curriculum, clinical education now begins in the first year, and students now see patients in week nine of their second year. This is a unique occurrence as very few university courses have their second-year students treating patients and taking responsibility for irreversible procedures.

The main reasons for this early clinical involvement are to facilitate greater opportunities for contextual learning and to improve the integration, balance and flow of basic and applied science material throughout the course. In the 'old' curriculum, these areas of learning were often not reinforced in the later years where the relevance would be more appreciated by the students. Students are now better able to apply their knowledge to practice, and they have improved clinical reasoning and communication skills. There is no doubt that students find the current course more stimulating and enjoyable and this all helps to promote lifelong learning and continued learning after graduation (Mullins *et al*; 2001b).

To help achieve these educational objectives, the new curriculum was designed as a small number of streams integrated both horizontally and vertically over the five years of the course (Figure 11.1).

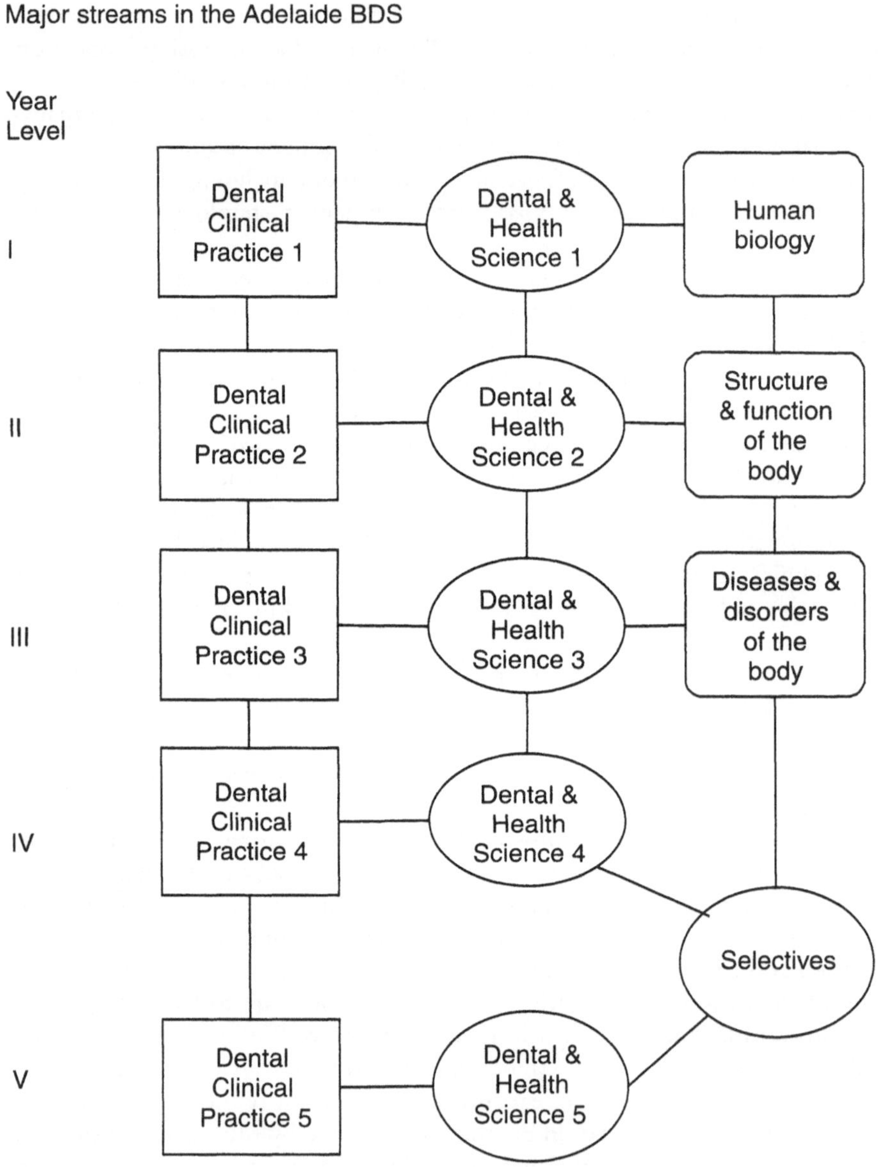

Figure 11.1 Curriculum structure of the Adelaide BDS

Students are introduced to clinical dental scenarios from day one of first year in the course 'Communication and Learning', which introduces them to what a dentist does in clinical practice (Greenwood *et al*, 1999). Their 'hands on' experience of many aspects of dentistry begins in their first year when they undertake tasks in the clinic that help them to become familiar and comfortable in working within the oral cavity, and within a multidisciplinary team. For example, by the end of first year they are able to:

- safely and accurately examine a patient and take a history;
- provide health recommendations on the basis of their analysis of a dietary history;
- recognize normal imaged structures and associated pathology on various types of radiographs;
- safely and effectively take dental impressions and analyse the resulting models;
- detect and diagnose dental plaque, caries, toothwear and staining;
- safely and accurately detect calculus and use scalers and curettes for simple scaling.

Dental Clinical Practice 2 is designed to build on the knowledge and skills students have acquired in their first year so that they can assess the dental health of selected patients and subsequently provide appropriate preventive, periodontal and simple restorative care as required. In addition to clinical experience, students also carry out laboratory exercises in order to learn the various methods and techniques and the use of common dental materials to restore teeth affected by dental caries. By the end of the first semester of Year 2 students achieve the following learning outcomes in the clinic. They are able to:

- demonstrate the different procedures required for the management of dental caries;
- demonstrate the handling procedures of the dental materials amalgam, composite resin and glass ionomer cements;
- demonstrate the technical skills of providing adhesive and small amalgam restorations of teeth on dental manikins and on natural teeth;
- use fluorides in the control of caries;
- assess the oral health of selected patients by using appropriate skills in:
  - communication;
  - history-taking;
  - clinical examination;
  - appropriate treatment planning;
  - recording and reporting.

In the third year, students carry out simple clinical procedures that require them to apply knowledge and skills acquired from Year 1 and Year 2 and from their formal classes to hospital patients. In the fourth and fifth years, there are two closely coordinated streams, Dental and Health Science and Dental Clinical Practice. In Dental Clinical Practice 4 and 5, students gain experience in more advanced aspects of clinical dentistry, including oral surgery, paedodontics, and fixed prosthodontics. During Year 5 students also do a two-week rotation to a rural practice and a metropolitan community practice.

By the end of Year 5 (their final year) students are expected to be able to carry out most of the functions of a professional dentist. To assist in the development of these skills, the class is divided into four 'practices' or 'firms' of 12 students each. Each practice consists of:

- a 'practice principal' who has both academic and clinical input into the group;
- a range of clinical tutors;
- a 'practice manager' who will ensure that the practice is busy and efficient;
- reception and dental assistant staff;
- students.

Within the practice students have the freedom (with guidance from the principal and within some operational constraints!) to plan their own strategies for achieving their treatment goals. This is a new concept beginning for the first time in 2001. It is envisaged that these 'firms' will eventually be expanded to embrace first to fourth year. Simple hygiene tasks will be performed by second and third year students, and patients will be referred within the 'firm' to fourth or fifth year students for more complex procedures. This will provide a more coherent treatment process for patients attending the clinic, and also an opportunity for liaison, and cross-age tutoring, between the different years of the course.

In medicine, similar curricular objectives and clinical outcomes can be identified. For example, objectives and learning outcomes at UWCM (1994) are specified in Table 11.1.

Table 11.1 Objectives and learning outcomes at the University of Wales College of Medicine

Objectives	**Level of Activity and Outcomes**
Year 1: to identify 10 key clinical features of normal cardiovascular function	examine patient in cardiology outpatients (OP) clinic or a surrogate patient; demonstrate features to clinical tutor
Year 2: to categorize the features (history and examination) of common cardiovascular disorders, eg stable and unstable angina	receive the history and examine for the cardiovascular pathology in appropriate patients in hospital or OP; discuss with medical house officer
Year 3: to consolidate and extend history and examination skills relating to the cardiovascular system linked to other systems	in the hospital, take a structured history and examination linking the organ systems, eg effects on locomotor, renal, ophthalmic systems of the cardiovascular disorder; present to colleagues and the medical team
Year 4: to learn how to explore the cardiovascular disorders in the contexts of past health, other systems, family and social situation	develop a rapport with the patient; relate symptoms and signs to the person in their family and social context; discuss with multidisciplinary members of hospital staff and medical colleagues
Year 5: to evaluate the clinical management of acute and chronic cardiovascular-based disorders	one-to-one attachment to a consultant with exposure to coronary care and diagnostic departments; draft treatment plan including post-hospital care involving multidisciplinary members of community team; agree plans with consultant

Irrespective of how clinical experience is integrated into the curriculum, in different MDV courses successful learning in this context depends on three critical factors:

- creation of a trusting environment;
- clinical practice being based on sound educational theory;
- introduction of a process of self-reflection and self-assessment.

Creating a trusting environment

Most students experience anxiety, and the clinical environment can be a daunting prospect. Often, they are performing unfamiliar tasks for the first time, and so it behoves us to create a productive learning environment so that the students feel free to express themselves, to question, to make errors, and not to be judged beyond redemption. Therefore, we need to formally develop an 'umbrella' of trust for the students. To help create this atmosphere, in small groups, we should encourage students to speak individually about themselves to the group so that a broader perspective is presented about each person. Encouraging humour and light-hearted openness helps to promote a trusting environment. Remember – learning can be fun!

Another method of helping to create a trusting environment is to ask students to make explicit their expectations of their clinical educators. The following list was produced in the first class meeting period at the start of fourth year oral diagnosis, after an overview of the year had been presented. A good tutor is one who:

- can empathize with students and communicate on the same level;
- demystifies the subject;
- criticizes without demoralizing;
- encourages by reinforcing the positives;
- is accessible out of hours for advice;
- allows you to determine the level you are at;
- keeps an open mind and will listen to alternative viewpoints;
- has a keen sense of humour;
- is patient;
- assesses students fairly.

This list then provided a set of criteria for the tutor's behaviour in the clinic (Wetherell and Mullins (1994). Students were also asked to develop their own objectives for the year in response to the question 'What do you want to be able to do at the end of the year that you can't do now?'. The resulting list was as follows:

- fifth year!;
- to be able to consider the patient as an individual and develop treatment to suit their needs;

- to have the ability to make a correct diagnosis;
- to be able to apply our acquired dental knowledge effectively;
- to acquire a holistic approach to treatment;
- to develop better communication skills with patients and tutors;
- to be able to work more effectively;
- to act on constructive criticism;
- to develop confidence in ourselves;
- to be able to take better radiographs;
- to be able to remain calm;
- to be able to develop a first-hand grasp of oral pathology;
- to have patience with patients;
- to develop complete organization.

These points helped students to focus their learning experiences in the clinic. The exercise also provided the opportunity for students to develop 'ownership' of their course and to feel empowered through having a direct input into the desired outcomes of their course.

To help promote a wider range of experiences, a session at the end of each clinical period was set aside to debrief as a group, and share each student's learning experiences. This was conducted in an open, friendly manner where students felt free to discuss and question each other about all aspects of their successes and failures. This approach provides a deeper learning pattern, as the reflective aspect of the Kolb learning cycle (see below) is being implemented immediately after the event. Feedback from the students indicated that these sessions were a very valuable part of the learning experience in the clinic, because students share their experiences with their peers, and learn from each other. These periods are best conducted in a room away from the clinic. Students must leave their 'egos' outside the door. This enables people to be less defensive about their mistakes and to be generally more relaxed and focussed about learning.

Similarly, in undergraduate medical teaching, there is increasing recognition that clinical skills, particularly history receiving, can take place in a trusting environment through observation (Dacre, 1998). Thus one student can take a history and be observed by a second student and a pre-registration house officer. The first student then observes the second student carrying out the clinical examination. Jointly the students present the case to the house officer who can respond through their knowledge of the specific patient, the clinical situation, and their observations of the history and examination skills. The students can then exchange roles for the next patient. This type of environment should be relatively safe for both students, and the situation is close to 'real' clinical experiences. However, it suffers from a lack of standardization and the student might be confused by the inter-house officer variations in history-taking and examining.

This approach can be extended to problem-based learning where a small group of five to six students see a patient on the ward under the guidance of a clinical tutor. They carry out an initial analysis and then they decide what further information they need, eg, literature on best evidence, retrieving tests results, investigating family and social issues, before presenting their diagnostic, treatment and further management plan on the 'whole person' to the tutor (Parikh, McReelis and Hodges, 2001). The advantages of this approach include crossing traditional medical disciplines, consideration of the home and social settings, analyses of the determinants of health, and feedback from the tutor. It is also a trusting environment as the students work together and they are not singled out for criticism. This approach can equally occur in primary care with a general practice tutor. Disadvantages include anxieties amongst the students about planning their own learning, difficulties in accessing the evidence, and the standardization of feedback from the tutors (Parikh *et al*, 2001).

The usefulness of formal educational theory

Learning in the clinic will be more effective if it is based on a sound philosophical view of learning – an example of the old adage: 'There's nothing as practical as a good theory!' When difficulties are encountered and changes are required for improvement, these can be related to the formal theory of learning rather than to the personality of the student or the tutor.

Kolb's cycle of learning

One such philosophical framework that we have found useful is that initially developed by Kolb (1984) (see Chapter 4 and Figure 4.4). Students arrive at the clinic knowing something about the tasks to be performed: they have 'grasped experience' from previous exposures, eg, in laboratory and clinical simulations. This 'abstract conceptualization' is elaborated by 'concrete experience' as the students work in the clinic. 'Reflective observation' can follow in seminar sessions after the clinic or in discussions with tutors, and will be extended and deepened in writing a journal of reflection (Wetherell and Mullins, 1996). The experience thus grasped by abstract conceptualization and concrete experience is transformed into knowledge by reflective observation.

This experience is also reflected upon during a self-assessment process at the end of each treatment session (see below). Formalizing the reflective process in journals or through self-assessment helps transform concrete experience into learning. As one student wrote: 'It is a good way to reflect on one's own experience and perhaps recognize where one's judgement or thinking was incorrect, and therefore perhaps learn from the situation. It allows one to recognize, in writing, the natural thought process.'

The 'active experimentation' phase is carried out in subsequent clinical sessions, thus completing the Kolb cycle. This provides students and staff with a theoretical framework within which to discuss student learning, and this assists both staff and students to focus on the central issue – how students learn.

Year 5 of the Wales medical curriculum provides an example of how links to the Kolb learning cycle can be clearly identified (University of Wales College of Medicine, 1994). The students have completed most of their final examinations and they are consolidating their general medicine, general surgery and general practice knowledge, skills and attitudes in preparation for their house officer year. The Secondary Referral Practice module lasts for eight weeks and each student is attached on a one-to-one basis with a consultant for four weeks of general surgery and four weeks of general medicine. The objectives include:

- verbalizing the assessment and management of acutely ill patients;
- defining reasons for admission (both elective and emergency) and for discharge;
- assessing the rational and efficient use of diagnostic and support services, etc.

Concrete experience

In the surgery attachment, attendance in the casualty department identifies cases and some are admitted and others discharged. The student follows admissions to the ward, to the operating theatre if surgical management occurs, to intensive care if necessary, back to the ward, and through rehabilitation to discharge or death.

Reflective observation

Students keep a self-assessment logbook that guides learning opportunities to help them to identify the breadth of experiences that they might encounter. A reflective journal is also kept to enable the depth of learning to be analysed. Discussions occur with the consultant about differential diagnoses, investigations, treatment and communications with the patient and family.

Abstract conceptualization

Formalization of the clinical learning occurs by written reports about a case and an area of personal, special interest. These analyses promote the linking of concepts of health, diseases, epidemiology, effectiveness of treatment et alia with the specific case. The case is presented to the consultant and others in the medical team and feedback is given.

Active experimentation

Students write a draft treatment plan with options for longer-term care. They can experience the patient's progress and observe the involvement of other hospital specialists and departments including operating, pathology and imaging. Their skills at intubation and vascular access can be developed, intensive care experiences demonstrate the maintenance of key systems in the critically ill, and their knowledge and attitudes about communicating with distressed relatives develop through real cases, etc.

Problem-based learning (PBL)

The other educational theory used in the Adelaide BDS is problem-based learning (PBL) (Mullins *et al*, 2001a). In the clinical arena, students are confronted by new problems each session. The educator's role is to guide students through the problem-solving process by asking appropriate questions. Within the trusting environment, students are therefore encouraged to take responsibility for their thoughts and actions. Students will discover what they know, but more importantly, what they don't know, hence an active learning experience is created.

All clinical sessions should provide a positive learning experience even if negative issues occur. In fact, these negative situations should always be turned around into positive learning issues. Some of the most valuable and long-lasting learning issues are generated by negative experiences. However, a constant awareness and monitoring of a student's anxiety is paramount, as anxiety impairs the learning experience.

Using a formal theory of learning helps provide a 'personality buffer' between tutor and student and the student undertakes responsibility for change because they understand what is required next time a similar situation arises. Therefore, personality differences between the tutor and the student are reduced, along with unnecessary negative anxiety. The journal of reflection also provides an insight into the student's personality and allows for a deeper understanding between student and teacher.

Self-assessment combined with open and precise criteria

Many clinical procedures performed are not obvious to the outside observer. For example, the only person who can critically appraise dental work is another dentist, and so it is vital that the undergraduate develops a keen awareness of what constitutes good dentistry. The work of medical and veterinary practitioners is more open to scrutiny, but the requirement to be critical of one's own performance applies just as much. As educators, we help mould our students by providing precise criteria of knowledge, skills and professional attitudes to allow the process of an accurate self-assessment to occur for all procedures. Student clinicians must learn all these skills during their five-year undergraduate years because on graduation this will be the only method available to judge their own performance.

One definition of self-assessment is the involvement of students in identifying standards and/or criteria to apply to their work and making judgements about the extent to which they meet these criteria and standards (Boud, 1996). Because we want our students to become lifelong learners, we must help develop a positive attitude towards, and skills in, self-assessment. We are educating the students in clinical practice to graduate from our institutions, with a vast array of skills and knowledge with the expectation that they are capable of regulating their own practice. To facilitate this process, we must actively involve our students in making judgements about their own standards of practice. Clear and precise criteria must be set, which both tutors and students use openly – no hidden agendas! If students are to become lifelong learners, they must develop excellent skills in self-assessment. There is very little point in having an assessment process merely to grade students. Assessment should primarily be about learning and students taking responsibility for that learning. Figure 11.2 indicates how the self-assessment process works in the Adelaide BDS (Wetherell, Mullins and Hirsch, 1999).

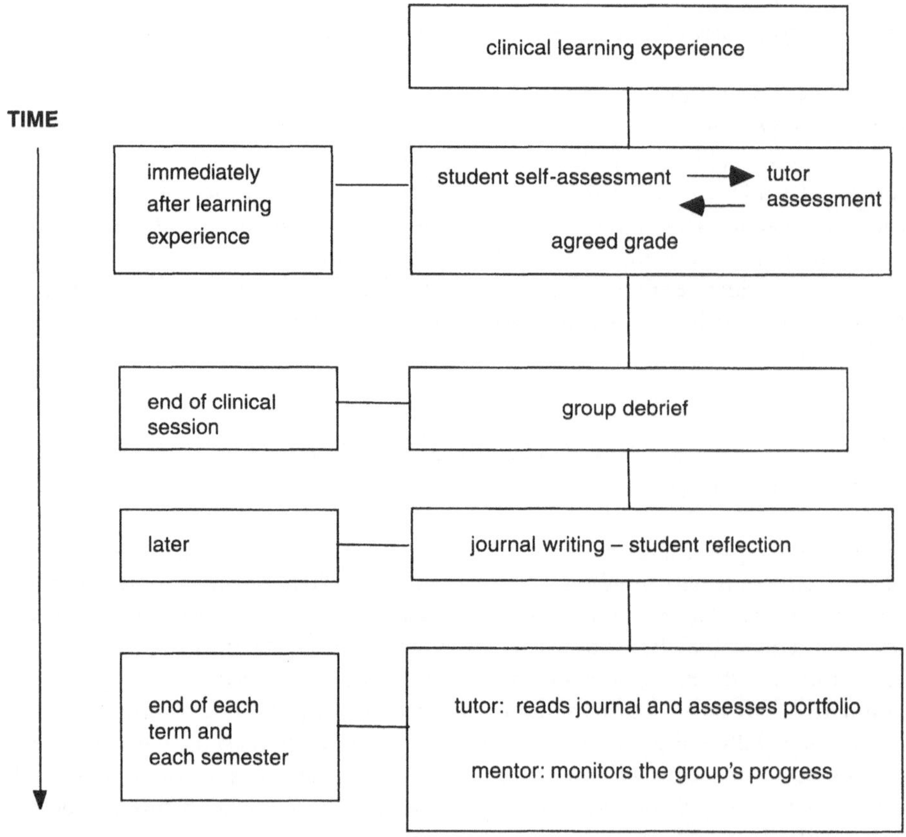

Figure 11.2 A flow-chart for self-assessment

The basic requirements of self-assessment are:

- **A clinical assessment criteria booklet**
  This provides, in detail, precise criteria for all clinical procedures and describes the requirements needed for excellent, good, satisfactory, borderline, and unsatisfactory grades. Both students and tutors have this booklet and it becomes the basis for self-assessment.
- **A self-assessment booklet**
  Each student is provided with a self-assessment booklet consisting of a pad, similar to a receipt book, containing about 100 sheets. On completion of a clinical procedure, the students assess their work in the self-assessment booklet, using the standardized criteria in the clinical assessment criteria booklet. The students then seek feedback from the tutor. The tutor's comments are also entered in the self-assessment booklet. If the tutor's assessment differs significantly from that of the student, the reasons are recorded during this process. A typical page from a student's pad is illustrated in Figure 11.3. The tutor removes the original and the student keeps the copy in the pad. Hence all assessments for each clinical discipline are retained as a permanent record by both the tutor and the student. This provides the staff mentor with an excellent overview of the student's progress.
- **Staff mentors**
  To assist in monitoring each student's performance, a staff mentor programme has been developed. Staff members are allocated six students for whom they are responsible for one year. The roles of the mentors are to:
  - assist students in obtaining and maintaining a group of patients appropriate to their needs, including the assignment, review, transfer and discharge of these patients;
  - assist students with difficulties;
  - review students' dental clinical practice assessment portfolios;
  - assist discipline and stream coordinators in determining mid-year and final grades.

  Mentors are expected to allow at least 30 minutes to meet each student to discuss their assessment portfolio each half-semester. The student is required to give a concise summary of the current treatment and what still needs to be done for each patient. The mentor must ensure that all aspects of the patient's health issues have been addressed in the treatment plan and that the treatment plans have been signed. They arrange for the discharge of patients who have finished treatment. The mentor reviews the number of patient treatments completed by the students, the pattern of patient attendances, and the student's record of self-assessment. They appraise the quality and quantity of the students' work in radiography, read and comment on students' journals of reflection, and request feedback about how any aspect of dental clinical practice could be improved. Students may seek a meeting with their mentor at other times for assistance with specific matters related to clinical practice. As a result of this process each student and mentor should have a precise understanding of the student's assessment status.

Student: John Smith		Year: 4	Mentor: Dr Wetherell
Patient: Mary Jones		Date: 10/9/01	Procedure: Relief of pain and access to the 14
	Student	Tutor	Learning issues
Infection control S/U	S	S	I need to be more careful in diagnosing pulpitis; sometimes pulp tissue is incompletely nonvital.
Knowledge base E/G/S/B/U	S	B	I need to revise access cavities for premolar teeth. This has been a good learning experience.
Skills E/G/S/B/U	B	U	I will write down what I would do next time in my journal.
Professional behaviour	Good		
Tutor's name: Dr B Black	Tutor's comments: The major learning issue was that you need to address the near perforation of the tooth when making your access cavity. I agree that you need to revise the design of access cavities. Signature: BB		

Figure 11.3 Clinical assessment pro-forma – Grades available S satisfactory; B borderline; U unsatisfactory; E excellent; G good

This uniform system of clinical assessment is intended to:

- give students direct input into their clinical assessment and learning experiences;
- standardize the assessment method from year to year and across the clinical disciplines;
- encourage students to reflect on the learning process as a whole;

- teach students to reflect on and assess the quality of their clinical work using a standardized clinical assessment procedure;
- encourage students to learn by receiving regular feedback;
- encourage students to accept responsibility for what they say and do in the clinic;
- introduce objective measures of clinical performance in each discipline;
- help develop lifelong learning skills.

Our understanding of how self-assessment works is illustrated in Figure 11.4. In the clinical setting, students are given the opportunity to identify the standard of their work against a set of criteria, and to take responsibility for the self-assessed grade. They are encouraged to reflect on their experiences, both immediately with the aid of their tutor, and later with the journal of reflection and their mentor. Therefore, a cycle for experiential learning is generated, the same Kolb cycle that is used to underpin student learning. The aim of this process is to establish good learning patterns that encourage the desire for lifelong learning through constant self-assessment.

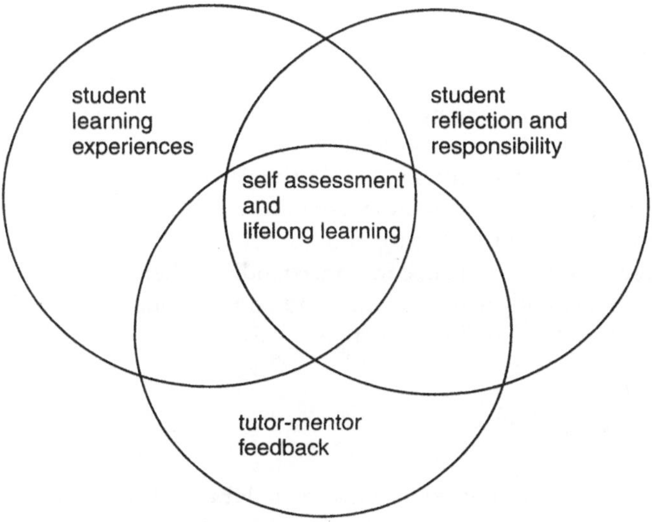

Figure 11.4 Self-assessment educational spheres of learning

Training for clinical tutors

In most MVD Schools, particularly in the later years of a course, there is a body of staff who act as clinical tutors for students working in clinics. At this stage of the course, students are preparing for independent practice and they need to gain clinical experience treating patients with a variety of problems. The function of tutors is to provide close supervision of students in a clinical situation rather than to teach in a classroom. However, it is important that they appreciate the philosophy and implementation of the curriculum within which the students have received their MVD education. This is particularly important if the tutors are part-time teachers, eg, postgraduate students or practitioners, who may have graduated from conventional and more didactic courses and may, therefore, not share the experiences of the new generation of students.

Clinical tutors, who will be working with students whose education has been within a PBL context, particularly require training to ensure that their approach to teaching is compatible with the students' experience. Without such training, tension and conflict tend to arise between tutors and students, the students' earlier educational experiences are devalued, and many of the benefits of PBL (confidence, self-evaluation, effective communication) may be lost. A training package for clinical tutors at the Adelaide Dental School consists of an introduction to the meaning, aims and values of PBL, and an explanation of the processes of a PBL session, again illustrated by a PBL scenario of a case of near collapse due to vasovagal syncope (Mullins *et al*, 2001a).

Conclusion

Clinical teaching is about giving and sharing, and provides us with a constant range of challenges to ensure our students have a safe and nurturing learning environment. Our own enthusiasm and interest in their progress acts as a positive catalyst for change. Embracing these essential principles will help produce a rewarding outcome for both educator and learner.

If we define learning as 'a change in understanding', then our role is to embrace this change by being enthusiastic, excited and compassionate – never forget your own frailties and really enjoy the challenge.

References

Boud, D (1996) *Implementing student self-assessment*, HERDSA Green Guide 5, Higher Education Research and Development Society of Australasia, Sydney

Dacre, J (1998) Clinical Work and Teaching, in *Medical Education in the Millennium*, eds B Jolly and L Rees, Oxford Medical, Oxford

General Medical Council (GMC) (1993) *Tomorrow's Doctors, Recommendations on Undergraduate Medical Education*, General Medical Council, London

Greenwood, F, Townsend, G, Joseph, V and Wetherell, J (1999) Introducing Adelaide dental students to a problem-based learning curriculum, *European Journal of Dental Education*, **3**, pp 15–19

Kolb, D A (1984) *Experiential learning experience as the source of learning and development*, Prentice-Hall, Englewood Cliffs

Mullins, G, Wetherell, J, Townsend, G, Winning, T and Greenwood, F (2001a) *Problem based learning in dentistry: The Adelaide experience*, Adelaide Dental School, University of Adelaide, Adelaide

Mullins, G, Wetherell, J, Townsend, G, Winning, T and Greenwood, F (2001b) Evaluating the curriculum of a PBL course, in *Problem based learning in dentistry: The Adelaide experience*, eds G Mullins *et al*, Adelaide Dental School, University of Adelaide, Adelaide

Parikh, A, McReelis, K and Hodges, B (2001) Student Feedback in Problem Based Learning: a Survey of 103 Final Year Students across Five Ontario Medical Schools, *Medical Education*, **35**, pp 632–36.

Townsend, G, Winning, T, Wetherell, J and Mullins, G (1997) New PBL dental curriculum at the University of Adelaide, *Journal of Dental Education*, **6**, pp 374–87

University of Wales College of Medicine (UWCM) (1994) *Integrated Medical Curriculum*, University of Wales College of Medicine, Cardiff

Wetherell, J and Mullins, G (1994) A problem-based approach to a course in oral diagnosis, *Australian Dental Journal*, **39**, pp 190–92

Wetherell, J and Mullins, G (1996) The use of student journals in problem-based learning, *Medical Education*, **30**, pp 105–11

Wetherell, J, Mullins, G and Hirsch, R (1999) Self-assessment in a problem-based learning curriculum in dentistry, *European Journal of Dental Education*, **3**, pp 97–105

12

Developing reflective clinical practice

Stephen Brigley

Introduction

The influence of reflective practice on professional education in the United Kingdom has grown remarkably since the 1970s. A host of initiatives, such as learning portfolios, reflective journals, diaries and professional mentoring schemes bear witness to its contemporary importance across the professions. Its impact in teaching, social work and healthcare has been widely studied and discussed. Prominent examples in the health professions include general practice (Al Shehri, 1995; Mathers *et al*, 1999; Brigley, 2001), public health medicine (Brigley *et al*, 1997b) and nursing (Ghaye and Lillyman, 2000). Portfolios, albeit with an assessment or regulatory purpose, have been adopted by some Medical Schools in the training of undergraduates, PRHOs (pre-registration house officers) and SHOs (senior house officers), and by the General Medical Council (GMC) in its proposals for the revalidation of doctors in the United Kingdom. It seems that reflective practice has achieved parity with apprenticeship and competence models of professional training (Furlong and Maynard, 1995).

To reflect means to engage in a deliberate act of thinking. Healthcare professionals obviously have to do this all the time in relation to clinical problems. The aims of this chapter are to help them understand and develop practical approaches to reflective practice. Strong opposition has been encountered to any form of 'navel gazing' (as reflection is sometimes called) from groups such as hospital consultants. For them, clinical effectiveness means gaining access to rational evidence and having the resources to apply it. Criticisms of reflective practice have also been voiced in nursing (Mackintosh, 1998) and in social work (Ixer, 1999). Even its advocates hold contrasting views of reflective practice, sometimes underpinned by differences of values and ideology (Moon, 1999a). This chapter will not engage with such debates, but it will begin by elaborating a theoretical perspective of reflective practice that is seen to be consonant with the practical methods and approaches that are its main concern.

A theoretical perspective

Reflective practice originated with Dewey (1933) who distinguished routine from reflective action. He conceived reflexivity as a state of mind, a way of problematizing professional practice that enables it to be shaped by autonomous judgement rather than the mechanistic repetition of set behaviours. Schon (1983; 1987) turned this into a radical vision of professional knowledge and competence and of how professionals learn and develop their practice. Drawing on studies of engineering, architecture and psychiatry, he highlighted the role of reflection in deliberative action: a stepping back from experience in order better to analyse and evaluate courses of action and determine how best to proceed. This form of reflection implies being able to take 'time out' to think freely, released from the pressure to make an immediate intervention. Schon contrasted this with reflection that takes place in action and is therefore not a separate, retrospective event, though arguably it requires some disengagement of the mind from the action (Eraut, 1995).

Dewey, by characterizing reflection as a state of mind, invites a holistic, inquiring posture towards practice. It may be likened to an attitude of mindfulness or attentiveness (Van Manen, 1991) by which professionals constantly regard their judgements as provisional and decisions as questionable and open to alternative interpretations. Mindfulness is necessary because of the conditions of uncertainty and diversity of values that pervade the contexts in which professionals have to make their judgements. A reflective professional is prepared when necessary to interrogate not only resources, methods and results but also fundamental goals, values and assumptions of practice.

To deliberate on alternative approaches to practice rather than accept one obvious answer, indeed to be generally inclined to do so, implies an openness to all options and a preparedness to subject them equally to critical interrogation. A patient's problem may be amenable to more than one diagnosis, or unexpected contingencies may force rapid revision of initial views of the problem. Thus, reflective practice implies a constant questioning of experience, entertaining alternative hypotheses, treating every solution as provisional, exploring clinical and social ramifications of decisions and generally maintaining critical self-monitoring of professional judgement and action. It is important that this critical, mindful quality of reflective practice extends to the professionals' evolving view of their overall social and moral mission.

The analysis of reflection thus far seems difficult to square with the notion of reflective skills. Professionals obviously reflect well or badly and with varying degrees of insight and relevance to practice. Dewey (1933) identified open-mindedness, wholeheartedness and responsibility as key reflective dispositions, resulting in a commitment that is personal as much as professional. But these do not equate with the calling up of a specific skill. Reflective skills will presumably be displayed in characteristic behaviours that can be taught, learnt and assessed in much the same way as other cognitive skills. Yet, to take one example, reflection by a hospital consultant on the care of a patient could take any number of forms: a quick discussion with a nurse, an entry in a personal journal, a search through a medical journal, etc. The possible manifestations of reflection are infinite, and none can be isolated as the correct performance consequent on the exercise of a skill. Indeed, the idea of framing a specific behavioural descriptor and predetermined standard seems incoherent here. How reflective activity is practised depends on the consultant's interpretation of the clinical case, the options for action and the availability of time for reflection. Reflective awareness is a way of thinking and relating generally to one's practice, providing the background to everything that passes for professional practice.

This opposition between reflective practice and competence models is reinforced by Schon's (1983) argument that means and ends are not separate in professional action. Reflective thinking brings together the goals of professional practice (for example, providing effective patient care) and methods (processes, relationships and strategies) that practitioners see as important in achieving them. It also implies a type of evidence that does more than support the skilful application of prepackaged knowledge. One view of professional expertise (Benner, 1984) suggests it is grounded in tacit knowledge that is difficult to separate out from what expert performers do. In order to uncover knowledge 'below the surface', research needs to be integrated with practice, not removed from it as an 'appliance of science'.

The view that knowledge is owned by professional academics and researchers and valued as a predictor of effectiveness reduces practitioners to a technical 'delivery' role. Schon's rejection of this technical-rational view of professional knowledge and practice has been politically useful in reaffirming the autonomy of professional judgement. His positive theses are less clear, however, referring to analogies between professional knowledge and craft knowledge, and between professional practice and artistry. Reflecting on practice is supposed to put practitioners in touch with the tacit knowledge that underpins their artistry, promising new levels of self-awareness, deeper understanding of professional experience, creative solutions to practice problems and enhancement of professional responsibility and collaboration.

Reflection, reason and intuition

Reflection appears to be a self-regulating function that ensures professional adaptability in the application of knowledge and skills to specific cases. However, it has also been suggested that professionals can also practise extended reflection, ie, thinking directed beyond their immediate professional sphere of influence. How this changes the quality of reflection may be illustrated by linking reflection to wider forms of professional cognition, including the awareness of professional values, personal commitments and interpersonal, affective aspects.

Reflection typically starts from some as an emotional, moral or intellectual response to experience (a thought, feeling, event or action). This arouses the professional's interest, perhaps producing a sense of discomfort that can activate various forms of knowledge, intuition and belief. A useful example is that of a nurse dealing with the enquiry of a terminally ill patient as to whether he or she is going to live (Rolfe, 2000). How does the nurse reflect in a way that supports his or her autonomous judgement and defensible professional action? Reference to the clinical facts is only one element of a judgement in this situation. Knowledge of the individual – what the patient might mean in asking the question – will play a key part. How the patient's words and behaviour are interpreted on this occasion may depend on the nurse's previous experiences of this person and similar cases. It may also draw on tacit or intuitive knowledge, ie, that accumulated from previous experiences and reflections on experiences, and generally enshrined in paradigm cases of terminal illness.

If the case requires instant reflection ('in action'), gestalt reactions may be triggered that draw on deep cognitive and affective structures in the nurse. Intuitive and experiential elements may be informed by wider bodies of knowledge such as principles of counselling, humanistic psychology and ethics. What results is a clinical judgement informed by 'knowledge of the patient's physical condition, psychological make-up and social situation' (Rolfe, 2000).

The exercise of professional judgement creates a distinctive form of evidence. The nurse's overriding aims and methods of achieving them in the above scenario are based not only in knowledge of experimental findings but also in the weighing of the beliefs and intentions of the participants. Clinical knowledge and expertise is customized to enable interpretations of and decisions on the clinical options in the light of affective and interpersonal aspects. The relating of clinical cases to their socio-emotional context is an incremental process from which 'informal' theory emerges (Rolfe, 2000).

Thus, reflection is one component of autonomous professional judgement, alongside clinical reasoning based in research evidence, academic knowledge, intuitive understanding and personal knowledge. But it can exercise a pre-eminent influence on the others through its generation of informal theories. The latter forms of evidence provide professionals with overview understandings and confidence in judgement because they have been gradually established through previous experience of cases in which knowledge, principles and beliefs have been synthesized in practice. It follows that informal theories are always tentative: they have to be open to further reflection and adaptation in the light of new cases. But, paradoxically, they help practitioners to feel secure and autonomous in making professional judgements in conditions of uncertainty.

Reasons to reflect on practice

The general claim that reflective practice is better practice is complex and not amenable to simple proof, but may involve some of the following related benefits:

- It involves professionals in actively constructing their self-understanding of practice problems.
- It increases awareness of self and of others.
- It enables underpinning knowledge and values to be adapted in various practice contexts.
- It can be used to convert all manner of professional experiences into meaningful learning.
- It supports practitioners in making autonomous judgements in conditions of uncertainty and values conflict.
- It assists the transition from novice to more advanced levels of professional expertise.
- It leads into meta-reflection and critical perspectives of knowledge and practice.
- It helps to sustain a commitment to self-directed and lifelong learning.

Reflecting on practice

General accounts of reflective practice may leave doctors with a sense that reflection is something elusive and mysterious: what exactly are health professionals doing when they reflect? Practical formats and studies of reflection indicate that it can contain a variety of forms and levels. (Al-Shehri, 1995; Brigley *et al*, 1997b). Moving from the simple reproduction of practice, a healthcare professional may reflect on minor corrections needed to fit performance and skills to the particular patient. A qualitatively different reflection occurs when confronted by incidents and events that challenge individuals' knowledge and abilities or even their concept of practice. Whereas we might expect a novice or trainee to acquire the first type of reflective capacity by observation and experience of working with senior colleagues, this is less likely in a critical incident. Deeper and more structured reflection on action, possibly in conjunction with colleagues, is important if the full implications for professional practice are to be drawn out of the event.

The uncovering of these implications in reflective writing usually entails composing a description of what is being reflected upon, coupled with some analytical and evaluative account of the subject. The following questions, designed for nurses to address critical incidents, will help to illustrate (Kenworthy and Redfern, 1998).

Description
What happened?
How were you involved?
What were your feelings at the time?

What specific contribution/interventions did you make?
What happened afterwards?

Analysis and evaluation
What were you trying to achieve?
Why did you intervene as you did?
What internal and external factors influenced your decision-making?
How could you have dealt with the situation differently?
What choices did you have to do things differently?
How do you feel now about this experience?
What have you learnt about yourself and how you deal with similar situations?
How could you use the learning from this exercise in your future practice?
Do you need to improve your knowledge and incorporate new objectives into your learning or action plan?

A reflective sequence of *describe–analyse–evaluate–plan further action* was used to assist the portfolio reflections of groups of general practitioners in Wales (Brigley, 2001). In this instance, it was applied not only to significant events but to other forms of learning and practice, such as personal reading, courses, audit findings and patients' problems. The following extracts are quoted to show something of the variety of aims and objects of reflection that may result.

Reflecting on a critical incident

Reflection on contact with the bereaved:

> It is said in life that only two things are certain: paying taxes and dying. I decided to concentrate on the latter.
>
> Some deaths are expected, some are a release of chronic suffering and ill health, others are accidental or completely without warning. All are a loss. Some families have good support; others may be less fortunate.
>
> The doctor may have been involved in care and could have prepared the family for the expected. At other times we are just there to answer questions, give advice or even to be a shoulder on which to vent anger or denial.
>
> I feel in our practice we have no routine plan of action that is followed when we learn of a death. Sometimes this is by fax or by a phone call or even by reading in the *Echo*. I know some practices send a card of condolence; others simply wait to be asked to call. We are somewhere in between… [*The doctor goes on to describe the death of a patient that led to further communications with the patient's widow…*]

I am not sure whether I should have treated her comments as an informal complaint or simply an information-gathering exercise. Whichever way, I had felt threatened, perhaps even a little humiliated, certainly it considerably dampened my enthusiasm for early contact with the bereaved, with the result our practice policy is not really much further advanced...

The breadth of reflection can be seen in the emphasis on emotions and interpersonal relationships that this case involves. Reflection on the clinical details of the case (not reproduced here) is evident in the description and review of the case and in generalizations to the practice as a whole in the portfolio entry. It links to practical reasoning that highlights the need for a bereavement policy, but tempered by a powerful emotional response to experience. The tone is philosophical: issues to do with death and dying evoke emotions and values that have to be worked through before the practice issue can be addressed.

Reflecting on practice in general

Critical incidents are not the only fertile stimuli to reflect. Indeed, a holistic view of reflection suggests that practitioners ought regularly to examine all aspects of practice and, if necessary, problematize clinical procedures that are generally accepted without question. The following is an example:

The ECG in general practice, underused or overused?

The practice owns an ECG machine and patients are referred in an irregular and unstructured way. Some for chest pains, some for palpitations and some for routine screening in newly diagnosed hypertensives.

I looked at this issue and decided that the place of the ECG in the management of the patient with chest pain is very limited and possibly dangerous. The diagnosis of ischaemic chest pain should be a clinical one and ECG used to confirm infarction or severe ischaemia only. It is established practice in secondary care to carry out three sequential ECGs before excluding myocardial infarction. A normal ECG in a patient with chest pain is meaningless and possibly lulls us into a false sense of security.

On the other hand, in diagnosing cardiac arrhythmias in the patient with palpitations and diagnosing left ventricular hypertrophy in the hypertensive is a very useful exercise.

Having badly deskilled in the interpretation of the ECG I have revised my basics and read *The ECG in Practice* by John R Hampton.

Reflecting on professional learning

Critical scrutiny of one's professional role may move reflection into meta-reflection, ie, the questioning of fundamental conditions or first principles that govern knowledge and values in clinical practice. Criticality that involves the appraisal of alternative perspectives, which can lead to thought turning back on itself; and critiquing modes of reflecting and knowing themselves. An example might be meta-reflection on the grounds for what generally passes as evidence in clinical practice or on what is meant by effective professional learning. In the following extract, a GP begins by reflecting on the practicalities of keeping a portfolio, then turns to what learning generally means to him:

> Looking back on my portfolio, I have become increasingly concerned that I have not been recording all my activities, significant events and cuttings. It is difficult to get into the habit of recording all the papers that I read in journals. Maybe I feel loathe to do this as critical appraisal is not a particularly favourite activity of mine. I have tried to address this issue by cutting out articles that I feel are important to me – that may alter the way I treat, investigate or address an issue that interests me or that may help educate me in a field I feel deficient in.
>
> To help me record significant events I now have a small notebook that I keep in my consulting room so that I can record events immediately. This will help me not just remember that the event happened, but also to help me address the issue rather than just forget about it as perhaps happened previously.
>
> I think that these activities are starting to alter the way that I think and act about learning, to make it much more meaningful and personally appropriate to me. I feel more enthusiastic about it and am not just 'points collecting'. This may not be reflected in this portfolio due to the initial poor record keeping but should be more complete in next year's portfolio.

Reflection on personal values, emotions and beliefs is an important complement to clinical and practical reasoning as key elements in changing practice (Boud, Keogh and Walker, 1985; Mezirow, 1991). Medical, dental and veterinary professionals aim to create socially and culturally valuable products. In an open, democratic society, professional values and attitudes should be instrumental in determining what those products are and how they are best achieved. Amid the inevitable diversity of value judgements on the purposes and functions of clinical and related educational practice, healthcare professionals need to set their clinical practice in a framework of personal values and attitudes. For them, reflective practice can help to promote personal awareness that embraces social goals and values and the conditions necessary for their achievement.

Building structured reflection

Reflection generally is demonstrated in writing. Reflective writing provides meaningful accounts of professional experiences, converting informal, practice-based learning (that otherwise may pass unrecorded and unanalysed) into public evidence of its occurrence, form and quality. Thus, it is a personal form of evidence, but one that can serve an accountability purpose. The writing grows out of the common experience of raising questions about a clinical matter, identifying problems, trying to solve them and applying the lessons to future situations. One benefit of writing has been identified as its strengthening of the linkage between reflection and subsequent planning or action (Brigley, 2001).

Practitioners usually need advice and support with reflective writing. Objects of reflection are legion, but the time and opportunity to reflect and write are often denied by countervailing service priorities. Attempts have been made to devise approaches, methods and formats that will capture more accurately and efficiently specific reflections on practice and learning (Moon, 1999b; Pietroni, 2001). Selectivity and focussing are essential, using structured learning and practice development frameworks such as personal learning plans. A focussed approach may help to reduce time management problems that are seen to arise from reflection on practice.

Reflecting from a long perspective

It is advisable at an early stage to review one's professional experience in both a wider and longer perspective. Reflecting on one's long-term aims in career and professional development can expand to take in movements within the speciality or profession as a whole, service, organizational or policy changes in the health sector and their interface with society. Thus, reflection is deepened by linking fundamental professional values to the political, social and moral bases of healthcare provision. In so doing, practitioners are engaging with their personal and professional identities. Reviewing one's curriculum vitae, for example, can bring into focus long-term professional achievements, responsibilities, aims and aspirations. The simple act of updating this professional record may trigger thoughts on one's professional situation, how fulfilling work feels currently or how it might be improved. The review may well evoke emotions and personal commitments, as well as professional concerns.

An alternative way to reflect on personal and professional wants and aspirations has been developed for nurses (Teasdale, 1996). Practitioners begin by plotting the directions and turning points of their life and career on a graphic 'river of life' design. This can be transformed into a timeline of the significant twists and turns of their clinical career. Further steps involve listing what they want from work and comparing their traits with those of close colleagues. This elaborates how they think of themselves, mapping their personal view of the world and of themselves within it.

Taking stock of life experience is another way of defining the self beyond mere professional roles. The elements that go to make up this personal, professional and career overview then are qualifications, work experience, non-work experience, what one wants from work, what one is like as a person. These overview reflections extend awareness of self in relation to professional aims, purposes and potentialities, and provide a framework for further reflections on practice.

The reflective cycle

Building on this framework-setting overview, specific reflections can be linked into a structured sequence of reflection points, analogous to the experiential learning cycle or audit process that is familiar in many healthcare settings.

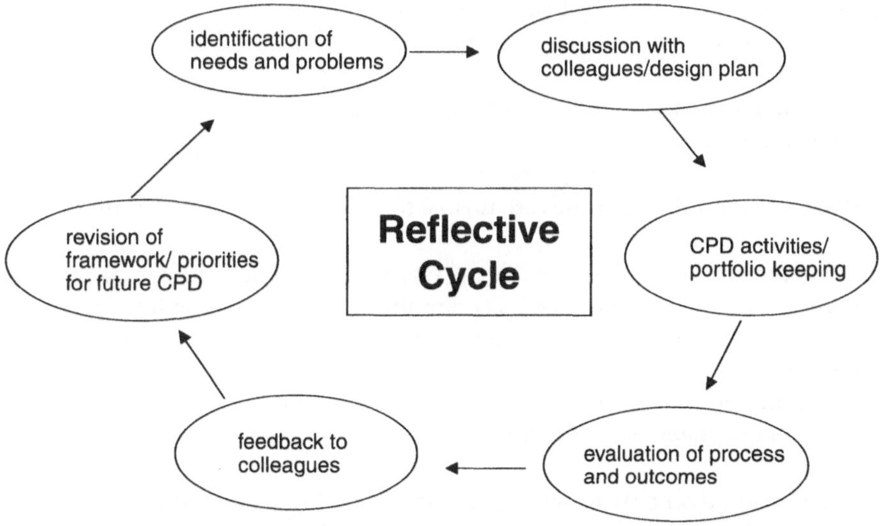

Figure 12.1 Reflective cycle (adpated from Brigley *et al* 1997a)

The cycle of reflection usually begins with some structured analysis of professional development needs, but appreciation of the role of different levels of reflection is unlikely to take root in this process without an explicit set of criteria to guide practitioners. To cite from a teacher development portfolio, it is expected that participants will demonstrate their application of various dimensions of reflection by:

- describing a teaching and learning situation or problem;
- selecting an appropriate principle or approach to apply to the problem;
- considering differences of process and outcome in relation to the implementation of particular teaching and learning aims or principles;
- analysing complex and multiple factors involved in an educational problem;

- evaluating wider implications of a particular strategy and consequences of applying it to a teaching and learning problem;
- showing awareness of alternative aims, strategies and contexts of teaching and learning and the ability to unite them in practice decisions;
- stepping back, critically reviewing and justifying fundamental aims, purposes and priorities in relation to education and its wider social context.

Application of the dimensions might involve a teacher in reflecting on professional development needs in a descriptive way:

> noting fluctuations in students' pass rates on MCQ (multiple-choice question) papers, student evaluations of sessions, modules or courses, records of teaching and lesson plans

Practice problems and significant events in teaching tend to encourage analysis and perhaps a closer focus on process:

> a PBL evaluation shows groups are unable to sustain self-directed learning

SWOT analyses, observational evidence (eg, videos of one's teaching), course review meetings, feedback from course committees and teams, ideas from personal reading, in-service courses and conferences and appraisal discussions also serve to promote analysis of options.

From identified needs, it is possible to frame CPD objectives. Sometimes these are put as general statements of method:

> 'need to read up on how to set MCQs' or 'ask colleagues how they facilitate PBL groups'

More specific behaviours or outcomes might be framed:

> should be able to set MCQ papers that reliably distinguish competence in 75 per cent or more of trainees taking college membership exams

> should have guided the group to be independent in access and use of learning resources within the first six months of running PBL tutorials

General and specific statements respectively involve different processes and levels of reflection and different types of learning. In the previous example, one line of reflection might focus on specific changes in methods of teaching or assessment. At another level, reflection might be on why the PBL students are having difficulty: whether autonomous learning is compatible with other elements of teaching, learning and assessment, with the approaches of some tutors or with the school experience and cultural expectations of the students. Reflection can help to bring a clearer and more precise understanding of the relevance of such issues, thereby opening up the possibility of action at a different level:

> a review of admissions criteria, PBL tutor support, a change of course objectives, new teaching or assessment strategies, etc

According to the interpretation of the problem, the strategies and methods suggested by these reflections could range from personal learning or in-service training aimed at having an optimal effect on the immediate situation, to collegial discussions of wider ramifications of the problem leading to institutional or professional action (group learning, joint projects, course reviews, action research, etc). These different understandings of the problem will be mirrored in contrasting approaches: the narrow focus on competence being more amenable to the measurement of learning attainment and practice outcomes, the broader strategy needing long-term inquiry and gathering of multilayered data on the impact of a group project.

Reflecting in portfolios

Reflections based mainly on reactions to practice problems can quickly become incoherent and fragmented. The portfolio is an all-embracing and flexible format that can overcome this drawback. It can be adapted to different purposes and stimulate reflection that is personal, professional and career-orientated. In essence, a portfolio is a collection of evidence of learning and professional development over time, evidence that in most cases is physically assembled in a loose-leaf, ring-bind file. Portfolios have to be distinguished from similar documents such as practice logs, records of achievement and performance profiles, which, while they also compile evidence, do not require reflective writing or related accounts of learning. A degree of personal choice of objectives and content, how these are organized, and over the subject matter and modes of reflection adopted are further distinctive features. As bad experiences of keeping portfolios have been seen to destroy a person's commitment to reflective practice, this chapter will end by tackling some key concerns.

An overarching issue is how structured the portfolio should be. A balance has to be struck in the portfolio between permitting reflective capacities to roam freely and providing guidelines that will maintain a professional practice focus. Portfolio guidelines vary in the degree to which they prescribe structure, contents and form of presentation. A less prescriptive format for a portfolio might consist of a list of topics or themes with light guidance on presentation, allowing participants to select 'found' items, reflective writing and contents that they view as related to the themes. This encourages the introduction of evidence and reflection on items that usually remain locked 'in their heads' or are passed over: spontaneous learning moments, minor adjustments of practice or new connections among concepts, facts and procedures. Reflection is more likely to encompass cultural expectations, implicit beliefs and theories that evoke collective understandings in the health professions and in society at large.

Prescriptive formats sometimes create a feeling of 'conforming to the rules' and diminish individuals' sense of ownership and creativity through the portfolio experience. Models and templates are increasingly used to help novice reflectors, but without prescribing any one in particular (Pietroni, 2001). However, these tools, indeed the reflective cycle itself, tend to be based on theories of adult and experiential learning, taking for granted a formula for reflecting that may not naturally fit clinical practice (Cornford, 2001; Eraut, 2001). Combining structured formats with selections from unstructured diary and journal entries (if necessary, labelled as 'private') is one way to safeguard a place for personal reflection. Even so, a semi-structured format of guiding questions for reflection (as, for example, on critical incidents above) seems preferable to reflecting against a checklist (a sure sign that reflection has been nullified).

Reflection is assisted if the aims of the portfolio are clearly and succinctly communicated to all involved. For example, two aims given to teachers for their portfolio are: to represent in a range of evidence the complexity and variety of a teacher's development over time – educational understandings, professional skills, moral insights and person knowledge; and to enable teachers to highlight teaching experiences that seem important to them and to show how these have been transformed into learning that is validated by personal reflection.

A further concern is how to encourage learners to reflect at more sophisticated levels. Using the dimensions of reflection above, there is a qualitative difference between reflection on a teaching problem that leads to the selection of an appropriate strategy and reflection that involves the weighing of alternative options and the justifications for each before deciding on the strategy.

Ideally, a portfolio should make the relationship of reflections, evidence, learning and practice transparent. However, it all takes time, not only to gain the skills of interweaving but also to gather adequate evidence and develop a longitudinal perspective on a complex activity such as teaching (probably a minimum of six months). The difficulty of representing these features in reflective writing has already been highlighted. Coherent links have to be built up between pieces of reflection and what is being reflected on (eg, descriptions of practice events, documents, or journal papers). Formats that allow limited physical space for exploratory writing will often stifle the kind of open-ended reflection that is needed, for example, to disentangle thoughts, ideas and emotions around a critical incident. Stipulation of the overall length of the portfolio, however, is probably justified, given the tendency of some to include numerous items of limited relevance and pages of random, ill-focussed musings. Portfolios ought to be biased towards quality rather than quantity. In the teacher development portfolio, abstracts, summaries and key pages with sections highlighted are to be included rather than whole reports and articles from general reading. The total length of the portfolio must not exceed 50 pages (not more than 25 pages of original writing and not more than 25 pages of additional materials).

Guidance on the structuring and presentation of the portfolio acts as an organizer, thereby stimulating further reflection. The guidance may suggest:

- A contents page.
- A written introduction of the content of the portfolio, its overriding aims and needs and any advice on how to read it.
- Dividers that clearly separate substantial sections, and headings that clearly distinguish reflection from other material.
- A written commentary on every 'found' item included in the portfolio.
- Brief summaries at the end of each section of insights gained by the participant.
- Ongoing personal reflections, building on professional development needs and expectations mapped out at the outset.
- A concluding section of written overview reflections on the portfolio and on professional growth that has taken place in the process of building it. Reference to the portfolio aims and criteria of reflection could provide important markers in this concluding evaluation.

Creative menus of alternative items for inclusion in the portfolio can add unusual dimensions to reflection. The addition of visual media or of creative writing, for example, may introduce new modes of symbolic and imaginative meaning and transform portfolio content. A menu of 'found' items and reflection points for teacher development is given below.

Section A	• relevant articles, reports, cuttings, communications and references;
	• notes, summaries, diagrams, charts, photos, drawings, poetry;
	• other performance evidence – eg, video, audio, electronic media productions, project reports;
	• session plans and materials, course documents, related publications produced by the learner.
Section B	• a learning plan, with objectives for teacher development defined and linked to strategies, resources and appropriate evaluation methods;
	• reflective accounts of learning activities, significant events and critical incidents;
	• extracts from a reflective diary or learning journal;
	• self-evaluations and evaluations of one's educational work by colleagues, supervisors, etc;
	• further analyses of personal learning needs and related plans for teacher development.

Figure 12.2 A menu of 'found' items and reflection points

The tendency of portfolios to become a mass of undifferentiated materials and ill-focussed writings can only be overcome by insisting that every item is accompanied by personal commentary and reflections and is cross-referenced to other items and entries. Those reflections, moreover, must address the fundamental aim of the portfolio, in the above example, by establishing the relevance of all items to the role of teacher or facilitator of learners.

Training and advice and, more crucially, peer support are probably essential to avoid the onset of atrophy in reflective practice. Ongoing dialogue with a circle of portfolios using colleagues produces insightful questions and feedback that maintain the momentum of reflection. Dialogues can be initiated in the informal talk of everyday teaching and clinical situations or in formal peer review, appraisal and mentoring interactions. Journal clubs, a long-standing forum for sharing professional interests, have been complemented by learning sets and workshops. These active, participatory and practice-based approaches give customized help to professional and interprofessional groups in reflecting on their experiences and views of practice (McGill and Beaty, 1992). Group reflection may be widened to include trainees and registrars, other health professionals, support staff and patients.

Conclusion

This chapter has been premised on the assumption that, with a basic understanding of the theory and of a method such as portfolios, everyone can make a start on reflective practice. It has had little to say on the deeper theory of reflection and group methods, concentrating instead on the concept of reflection, a normative view linked to other forms of knowledge and expertise, examples of various dimensions and levels of reflection and the portfolio approach to reflection for purposes of self-directed learning and professional development.

I am grateful to Cindy Johnson (University of Wales College of Medicine) and to one of the editors for comments on an earlier draft of this chapter.

References

Al-Shehri, A (1995) Learning by reflection in general practice: a study report, *Education for General Practice*, **7**, pp 237–48

Benner P, (1984) *From Novice to Expert. Excellence and Power in Clinical Nursing and Practice*, Addison Wesley Publishing Company, Menloe Park, California

Boud, D, Keogh, R and Walker, D (1985), *Reflection: turning experience into learning*, Kogan Page, London

Brigley, S, Littlejohns, P, McEwen, J and Young, Y (1997a) Continuing Education for Medical Professionals: a Reflective Model, *Postgraduate Medical Journal*, **73**, pp 23–26

Brigley, S, Littlejohns, P, McEwen, J, and Young, Y (1997b) *An Evaluation of the Pilot Continuing Professional Development Diary*, Faculty of Public Health Medicine, London

Brigley, S (2001) *Portfolio Learning among Groups of General Practitioners in Wales: a pilot project*, Occasional Paper Series, School of Postgraduate Medical and Dental Education, University of Wales College of Medicine, Cardiff

Cornford, C (2001) The development of practice professional development plans from the postgraduate educational allowance: a discussion of the causes and implications, *Medical Education*, **35**, pp 43–48

Dewey, J (1933) *How We Think – a Restatement of the Relation of Reflective Thinking to the Educative Process*, Heath, Boston

Eraut, M (1995) Schon Shock: a case for reframing reflection-in-action?, *Teachers and Teaching: theory and practice*, **1**, pp 9–22

Eraut, M (2001) Do continuing professional development models promote one-dimensional learning?, *Medical Education*, **35**, pp 8–11

Furlong, J and Maynard, T (1995) *Mentoring student teachers: The growth of professional knowledge*, Routledge, London

Ghaye, T and Lillyman, S (2000) *Reflection: Principles and practice for healthcare professionals*, The Cromwell Press, Trowbridge

Ixer, G (1999) There's No Such Thing As Reflection, *British Journal of Social Work*, **29**, pp 513–27

Kenworthy, N and Redfern, L (1998) *The Churchill Livingstone Professional Portfolio*, Churchill Livingstone, London

Mackintosh, C (1998) Reflection: a flawed strategy for the nursing profession, *Nurse Education Today*, **18**, pp 553–57

Mathers, N, Challis, M, Howe, C and Field, N (1999) Portfolios in continuing medical education – effective and efficient?, *Medical Education*, **33**, pp 523–30

McGill, I and Beaty, L (1992) *Action Learning Sets*, Kogan Page, London

Mezirow, J (1991) *Transformative dimensions of adult learning*, Jossey-Bass, San Francisco

Moon, J (1999a) *Reflection in Learning and Professional Development: Theory and Practice*, Kogan Page, London

Moon, J (1999b) *Learning Journals: A handbook for academics, students and professional development*, Kogan Page, London

Pietroni, R (2001) *The Toolbox for Portfolio Development: A practical guide for the primary care team*, Radcliffe Medical Press, Oxford

Rolfe, G (2000) *Nursing Praxis and the Reflective Practitioner*, Collected Paper Series, Nursing Praxis International, London

Schon, D (1983) *The ReflectivePractitioner: How professionals think in action*, Basic Books, New York

Schon, D (1987) *Educating the Reflective Practitioner: Towards a new design for teaching and learning in the professions*, Jossey-Bass, San Francisco

Teasdale, K (ed) (1996) *Mosby's Personal Professional Profile*, Times Mirror International Publishers Ltd, London

Van Manen, M (1991) *The Tact of Teaching*, The State of New York Press, New York

13

Drawing together quality issues, institutional benchmarking and revalidation

Iain Robbé

Introduction

The importance of high-quality teaching in our medical, dental and veterinary vocations is increasing. In this chapter, I shall discuss the stimuli for quality in teaching, issues around the governance of teaching, and the experiences of using a checklist as a practical way to promote quality for our needs and the needs of the various institutions. In the context of this chapter, you might be a teacher employed by a university or institute with separate responsibilities for research and/or clinical practice, or a teacher from a general or specialist practice with sessions for teaching via an honorary contract.

Quality

For a working definition, I am using quality as a broad term to describe the extent to which a teaching activity achieves what it is planned to achieve. The basic level of quality assessment is to measure the inputs, processes and outputs of teaching against the standards specified for each and to improve on the results (Elton, 1998), although it is widely recognized that measuring teaching quality is highly contentious, and rewarding teaching quality is equally disputed (McLean, 2001).

However, the experiences from hospital reforms that have tried to increase the focus on outcomes and quality have identified the willingness of professional groups to respond positively if they are involved in developing valid and reliable data as well as seeing bottom-up cultural changes (Ayres, Wright and Donaldson, 1998; Degeling, Kennedy and Hill, 1998).

The stimuli for quality in teaching

Medical, dental and veterinary professionals have a sense of vocation that is similar to other professionals (Dahrendorff, 1984). However, we are also similar to humans in general with regard to our needs and Maslow's hierarchy (cited in Curzon, 1990) is relevant when considering our needs and quality in our teaching (see Figure 13.1).

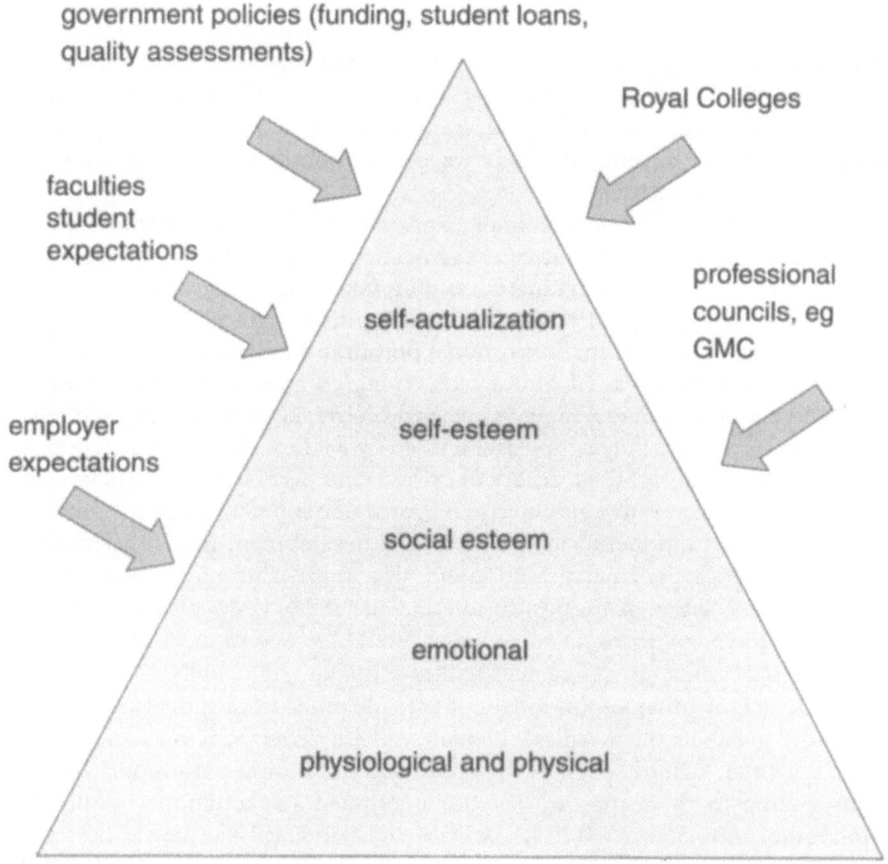

Figure 13.1 Diagrammatic representation of the external influences on teachers' needs

At the base of the pyramid, the teachers' physiological and physical needs must be met so the work environment should provide sufficient remuneration for survival. The infrastructure should include access to information on best evidence, other education technology should be available, and there should be time to plan.

Then the emotional and social needs must be met so the teachers should have empathic colleagues in the education setting, thus minimizing the pressures from inappropriate competitiveness. There should be a close alignment of objectives between departments and it should be easy to form alliances and partnerships so that collaborative teaching can occur. The adult learners, the employers and society at large should value the roles of teachers.

The next level of the hierarchy is for self-esteem and so the teachers should receive attention and recognition of their contributions. Their leaders should be empathic and supportive of our learning needs and continued development. It should be safe for us to promote innovative learning and not to be fearful of failure.

Finally there is the peak of the pyramid when self-actualization or fulfilment occurs and I would suggest that as professionals with our sense of vocation, we are motivated for the highest self-actualization. This need will be met if we can identify explicitly that our teaching practices promote and achieve the student learning that we are aiming for, ie, if we can demonstrate that our practices produce high-quality teaching.

We are also conscious of the increasing expectations of our student learners and the associated demands with students facing increasing debts while they are undergraduates and with postgraduates needing quality teaching to enable them to keep up to date (Elton, 1998). In between our own motivations and the learners' demands, there are the institutional pressures on quality. Our employers are responsible for the appraisal of our work using comparative data from local, regional and national sources. There is a major problem about the validity and reliability of data on quality in teaching as discussed by McLean (2001). For example, how are the judgements of the learners, peers and employers weighted and linked, and how are long-term outcomes such as personal development to be measured?

Appraisal is also supposed to identify personal development needs that should be translated into a personal development (learning) plan and if the plan is achieved then the learners, the institution and the individual would all benefit. Furthermore, the information from appraisal should be used to meet the requirements for our revalidation (General Medical Council, 2000) with the General Medical, Dental, or other professional councils. Another institutional tier that is pressing for quality is the Medical, Dental and Veterinary Royal Colleges and faculties with the various schemes for audit and continuing professional development leading to their approval for our continued accreditation (Faculty of Public Health Medicine, 2000). The policies and standards that are set by these bodies should be consistent with the expectations and activities of the majority of practising professionals. A further institutional stimulus for quality comes from the government policies for improvements in professional practices exemplified in the

National Health Service (NHS) since the election of the Labour government in 1997 by the clinical governance initiative (Secretary of State for Health, 1998). Governance is defined broadly as 'a framework through which NHS organizations are accountable for continuously improving the quality of their services and safeguarding high standards of care' (Secretary of State for Health, 1998) and the employer has the responsibility for the governance. Many teaching activities take place in NHS organizations, many of us hold honorary contracts with the NHS and it seems reasonable to accept that the issue of governance applies to teaching. A working definition would be that teaching governance is a framework through which teaching organizations are accountable for continuously improving the quality of their teaching and safeguarding high standards of education.

Other government policies arise from expert reports. For example, the *Dearing Report* (Department of Education, 1997) recommended a continuation audit of teaching quality that would evaluate the validity, reliability and sufficiency of teaching programmes. In summary, the stimuli for high-quality teaching include:

- our own self-motivations;
- the expectations of our learners;
- the institutions like the Royal Colleges who are responsible for our continued accreditation;
- the statutory regulatory councils who are responsible for our revalidation;
- employers who are responsible for the appraisal processes and for implementing the government policies.

The next section in this chapter explores governance in teaching.

Issues in the governance of teaching

In order to improve teaching quality there should be regular evaluating of outcomes by measurements with high validity and reliability but there are few standardized measures (McLean, 2001) and there is little systematic evaluation (Elton, 1998). However, these measures could be developed if they were part of a 'teaching quality strategy' in a governance framework. It is possible to adapt the clinical governance literature (Ayres, Wright and Donaldson, 1998; Paris and McKeown, 1999) to the teaching settings and I would argue that our institutions would be promoting teaching quality if they had:

- clear lines of responsibility for the overall quality of teaching and a structure that identifies a lead, eg, vice-dean (teaching) at the same level as the vice-dean (research) with both reporting to the dean/provost;
- teaching quality strategies with improvement processes, eg, one-to-one peer review, mentors, audit, that are linked to the other quality improvement processes in the institution, eg, research, clinical, human resources;

- explicit policies to identify good practices locally, regionally and nationally with innovations and evaluations to disseminate them;
- systematic collection of data on teaching quality; the data having high validity and reliability to monitor teaching and the achievement of appropriate standards;
- clear procedures to identify poor quality teaching at an early stage with constructive remedies to prevent negative effects on the learners;
- all personal development (learning) plans based on individual needs with the plans reflecting the principles of continuously improving teaching quality.

I have identified many of the stimuli in support of quality teaching and I have argued that measurements alone, even if they could be identified and standardized to achieve a broad measure of professional support, would not be sufficient to raise standards without a teaching quality strategy. Also, a strategy needs a governance framework through which teaching organizations are accountable for continuously improving the quality of their teaching and safeguarding high standards of care. The next section discusses how teaching governance can be taken forward.

A checklist to promote quality teaching

There are a number of common themes in the medical literature about the concepts of governance (Paris and McKeown, 1999; Scally and Donaldson, 1998) and I have developed a checklist based on the hypothesis that if these themes could be measured and if they were found to be positive then the concepts of governance could become more specific. The purpose of including the checklist here, in the case study below, is to suggest that it could be useful in your teaching setting for the development of the teaching governance framework and strategy based on the items identified in this chapter under the heading 'Issues in the governance of teaching'. These developments will require cultural changes in your institutions (Ayres, Wright and Donaldson, 1998) and the production of values and ground rules to facilitate individual participation (Paris and McKeown, 1999).

A case study

Background

In a lunchtime meeting, 10 postgraduate teachers in a medical college volunteered to participate in a pilot of the checklist. They were not a representative sample of teachers and they were approached because of their attendance at the monthly journal club lunchtime meetings. They were told that their responses were confidential but they were asked to discuss their responses at the meeting in terms of the checklist's validity (Cohen and Manion, 1989) compared to the literature, their experiences and governance issues. I facilitated the use of the checklist and the consequent discussion.

CHECKLIST

This checklist contains a series of questions for you as an individual with the responses confidential to you. You might want to respond to the questions and to write comments in the free text spaces.

1. Please identify one specific task you are trying to achieve as a professional teacher – maybe today, this month, this year…	The rationale for this question is that I wanted the participants to base their thoughts on quality in a specific context. Was the one thing, for example, an objective in a lesson plan about increasing knowledge or altering attitudes or acquiring a psychomotor skill? Was it about designing a teaching session or a new course or a new assessment process?

Free text space for comments:

The essence of this question is the fact that if I cannot identify a specific task that I am trying to achieve as a teacher then how can I assess its quality?

2. How would you evaluate the infrastructure in your department to support or facilitate your professional practice for that specific task?	The rationale for this question is that I wanted the participants to assess the infrastructure available to them. This is in terms of information, access to sources of best education evidence, time to plan, the appropriateness of education technology, et alia.

highly supportive	**supportive**	**average**	**unsupportive**	**highly unsupportive**

Free text space for comments:

The essence of this question is the fact that if I cannot identify a specific task that I am trying to achieve as a teacher then how can I assess its quality?

3. How would you evaluate coherence in your teaching department? I defined coherence as the amount of consistency between individuals and groups, and it is concerned with the amount of contact between people for shared purposes.	The rationale for this question is that I wanted the participants to evaluate coherence issues. These could be expressed in terms of objectives between individuals in a team, group, unit, eg teaching versus research versus clinical practice; is there a close alignment of goals as expressed in different department plans? Communication – do people talk easily in corridors and offices, do e-mails and memos flow between people or do they have to pass via section and department heads? Are there alliances and partnerships?

highly coherent	**coherent**	**average**	**incoherent**	**highly incoherent**

Free text space for comments:

The essence of this question is the fact that if I cannot identify a specific task that I am trying to achieve as a teacher then how can I assess its quality?

4. How would you evaluate the cultural issues for your teaching practices generally within your department?	The rationale for this question is that I wanted the participants to assess the openness of their departmental culture. Consider whether the culture is participative and open or closed off; is the leadership empathic and supportive? Is there a commitment to continued professional development with an accessible training budget? Is constructive questioning encouraged? Generally, is there teamwork or are individuals competing?

highly participative	**participative**	**average**	**unparticipative**	**highly unparticipative**

Free text space for comments:

The essence of this question is the fact that if I cannot identify a specific task that I am trying to achieve as a teacher then how can I assess its quality?

5. How appropriate are the teaching tasks that you wish to carry out (or, have to carry out) in the light of your training and competencies?	The rationale for this question is that I wanted the participants to assess the risks in their teaching. Were they asked to carry out tasks beyond their training and competencies? Could they be innovative? Did they have clear remits and task definitions? Were there commonly accepted standards for the tasks they have to perform?

highly appropriate	**appropriate**	**average**	**inappropriate**	**highly inappropriate**

Free text space for comments:

The essence of this question is the fact that if I cannot identify a specific task that I am trying to achieve as a teacher then how can I assess its quality?

6. How well developed are any systems for you to assess your performance?	The rationale for this question is that I wanted the participants to reflect on the assessment of their performance. Was there effective self-regulation? Were there systems for feedback from colleagues and if there were, how were they organized and did they have high validity? Were there systems for the early recognition of difficulties in delivering teaching and were there sensitive, constructive remedies to help overcome the difficulties?

highly developed	**developed**	**average**	**undeveloped**	**highly undeveloped**

Free text space for comments:

The essence of this question is the fact that if I cannot identify a specific task that I am trying to achieve as a teacher then how can I assess its quality?

Results: validity

The respondents easily identified tasks they aimed to achieve to provide high-quality teaching. The issues of infrastructure, coherence, culture, appropriateness of tasks, and systems to assess performance were evaluated average, positively or highly positively. In terms of content validity, the respondents considered that the checklist covered the concepts and characteristics of governance in teaching as far as they are known, both comprehensively and in a balanced way. However, they said it was not possible to answer the questions without the oral guidance from me so there are issues about intergroup reliability if my guidance was not standardized.

In terms of construct validity, there was a correlation between related variables, eg, a highly supportive infrastructure and a highly participative culture, and average or appropriate tasks correlated with average or developed systems to assess performance. There were no negative responses. On balance therefore, we concluded as a group that the checklist had moderate to high content and construct validity.

Results: evaluation of responses

It was important to focus the evaluations at a group level that was close to the respondents, ie, at the section or department level rather than at school of postgraduate studies or college level, as there were too many variables at the higher levels. The context of a specific teaching task was helpful and none of the respondents judged the infrastructure to be unsupportive. However, if there were difficulties with the infrastructure issues then these could be discussed constructively at the time of the annual appraisal. The developing new systems for revalidation and continued accreditation are intended to be informed by appraisal issues so if there were infrastructure difficulties then these should not be attributed to an individual but to a higher level.

There were high evaluations of coherence issues at the section and department levels with alignments of goals based on the annual plans. Thus alliances and collaborations were easy for informal advice and sharing of ideas as well as more formally, eg for teaching sessions, and for teaching research proposals. If there had been weaknesses of coherence with plans and goals then these could be discussed at section or department meetings.

The culture was participative and the appraisal forms required a continuing professional development plan to be written. This attention on the individuals' development helped their self-esteem needs and also it enabled the plans for their further contributions to receive attention and recognition.

Most teaching tasks that had to be undertaken were appropriate and the positive culture and coherence of goals encouraged innovations without a pronounced fear of failure. Anecdotally, there was an awareness that in other schools, teachers were sometimes given tasks beyond their training. It appeared to be difficult to achieve quality teaching practices under these circumstances and the professional medical, dental and veterinary cultures do not encourage people to admit to weaknesses or to a relative lack of competence. Ideally the appraisal processes should identify inappropriate tasks, consequential risks and learning needs.

Generally there were acknowledged notions about what quality teaching meant in different contexts and individuals could judge the extent that they achieved high quality. Usually the teachers were self-regulating, although feedback from colleagues was available. However, the systems for feedback appear to be largely informal and there are opportunities to develop systematic processes to assess performances with high validity and reliability and people will need to be trained to carry out these assessments. A recurrent theme was that an individual teacher could only carry out quality assessments to a limited extent. The respondents considered that the immediate grouping, eg, section or department, has a key role in finding the infrastructure resources, promoting coherence issues, creating a culture of collaborations and partnerships, and agreeing appropriate tasks and personal development plans. The higher organization, eg, university or institute, has to respond to the sections and departments by relating the issues to the external influences, eg, the government and the regulatory bodies.

Conclusions

We recognized that the 10 respondents were enthusiasts and their judgements might not be representative of other postgraduate teachers in the college. Further research is needed to test the validity and reliability of these results with medical, dental, veterinary and other professional teachers of undergraduates and postgraduates. You might want to use the questionnaire in your teaching department and I would welcome any feedback to me via the contributors' address at the front of this book.

The primary reason for developing the questions in the checklist was to make the issues of quality, particularly the links to teaching governance and institutional benchmarking of standards and outcomes, more specific. Setting aside the problems concerning the validity of quality measures in teaching, arbitrary measurements of quality will not benefit our students or ourselves if the measurements are not part of a teaching quality strategy including a governance framework. I suggest that the checklist is a method for making the governance issues explicit so that any appraisal of our teaching quality is in the context of the governance framework.

Conclusion

There are many stimuli for quality in our teaching, and assessments of quality need to occur within a teaching quality strategy and a governance framework. The checklist is proposed as an effective way to take forward the strategy and governance issues. Our employers in tertiary and continuing education are responsible for working with us to set up the strategy and framework based on explicit values, improvement processes, valid benchmarking data, and personal development plans. The employers are also responsible for setting up mutually beneficial appraisal systems that will contribute to our continued accreditation by the Royal Colleges and to our revalidation by the statutory regulatory councils.

References

Ayres, P J, Wright, J and Donaldson, L J (1998) Achieving Clinical Effectiveness: the New World of Clinical Governance, *Clinician in Management*, **7**, pp 106–11

Cohen, L and Manion, L (1989) *Research Methods in Education*, 3rd edn, London, Routledge

Curzon, L B (1990) *Teaching in Further Education*, 4th edn, Cassell Education, London

Dahrendorff, R (1984) In Defence of the English Professions, *Journal of the Royal Society of Medicine*, **77**, pp 178–85.

Degeling, P, Kennedy, J and Hill, M (1998) Do Professional Subcultures Set the Limits of Hospital Reform?, *Clinician in Management*, **7**, pp 89–98

Department of Education (1997) *Higher Education in the Learning Society (Dearing Report)*, Department of Education, London

Elton, L (1998) Staff Development and the Quality of Teaching, in eds B Jolly and L Rees, *Medical Education in the Millennium*, Oxford Medical, Oxford

Faculty of Public Health Medicine (2000) *Good Public Health Practice. Standards for Specialists in Public Health*, Faculty of Public Health Medicine, London

General Medical Council (2000) *Revalidating Doctors. Ensuring Standards, Securing the Future*, General Medical Council, London

McLean, M (2001) Rewarding Teaching Excellence. Can We Measure Teaching Excellence? Who Should Be The Judge?, *Medical Teacher*, **23**, pp 6–11

Paris, J A G and McKeown, K M (1999) Clinical Governance for Public Health Professionals, *Journal of Public Health Medicine*, **21** (4), pp 430–34

Scally, G and Donaldson, L J (1998) Clinical Governance and the Drive for Quality Improvement in the New NHS in England, *British Medical Journal*, **317**, pp 61–65

Secretary of State for Health (1998) *The New NHS, a First Class Service*, HMSO, Department of Health, London

14

The way ahead for medical, dental and veterinary education

Heather Fry and Sharon Huttly

Introduction

The education of medical, dental and veterinary (MDV) professionals has changed rapidly in recent years. Influences for change have come from many directions. These include changes in higher education (such as abolition of the student grant in the 1990s) and in higher training (eg, the Calman Reforms to higher specialist training in medicine). Another factor is the changed attitude of the general public to health professionals and the care they expect. Changed patterns of delivery of care, 'high tech' interventions, and solutions that are enormously costly, coupled (arguably) with insufficient resources for healthcare and education, have added to the complexity of the picture. Expansion of numbers of clinicians in at least one of the three areas and the restructuring of grades within these professions (and related ones) are also having an impact. These changes, and many others, are part of the new environment in which those who educate and train, work. The changes have profound implications for the practice of teaching, for assessing and designing curricula, and for learning.

The earlier chapters of this book largely focus on a single key theme, method or arena for teaching and learning, and largely on undergraduate education. This chapter takes a more inclusive approach and attempts to weave together several of these discrete themes, set them against some of the changes mentioned above and use this as a way of highlighting where education for the three subjects and professions is likely to focus in the years ahead.

The authors base their overview on their understanding of pedagogic processes and on the changes alluded to above. These are used in combination with key documents. The four main documents used with respect to the undergraduate years were *Tomorrow's Doctors* (GMC, 1993) and its draft supplement (GMC, 2001); *The First Five Years* (GDC, 1997), and; the *Framework for 2010 and Beyond* (RCVS, 2001). For post-registration education the documents most heavily drawn upon were *Lifelong Learning* (GDC, 2002); the *Duties of a Doctor* (GMC, 1995); information on the GMC Web site [http://www.gmc-uk.org/revalidation/index.html]; and the *Framework* (RCVS, 2001). One preliminary conclusion highlighted by these documents is that where medicine treads today, the other two professions may tread tomorrow. This is not to say that medicine has nothing to learn from the other professions; it has much. Nor is it to say that the training needs and solutions of each profession are identical. For example, a notable difference between medicine and the other two is in respect of the level of practical competence and independent practice expected upon university graduation.

In looking to the future of MDV education, we address three principal themes: integrated pedagogy for practice; professional practice; and lifelong learning.

Integrated pedagogy for practice

Designing curricula for learning

Chapters earlier in this volume have drawn attention to various facets of the teaching and learning process, including teaching and learning in and from different settings, such as the lecture theatre or clinic/ward/surgery, using IT, types of assessment, etc. An important task for the reflective – and effective – teacher is to consider how these all fit together. This task is important within sessions, even more important for a unit/course/module and essential at the level of the whole curriculum. For example, what are the most appropriate forms of assessment for a problem-based learning course and are they the same as those best suited to a lecture course?

Where transmission is seen as the primary teaching task and reception as the primary task of learners, approaches to teaching, learning and assessment may be congruent, but they will be limited. The tendency with such a view is to transmit and then test recall of pure content. A mismatch of method and desired outcome is a key part of the 'transition' problem that may still occur in the evolution from the early years of training to the later. Methods of teaching may, or may not, become more elaborated (for reasons of fashion, evidence-based pedagogy or regulation), without assessment or notions of learning keeping pace.

How then may curriculum design, teaching methods, conceptions of and approaches to learning and modes of assessment be selected for the task in hand, be congruent with it, and aligned with each other? A threefold approach will ensure some degree of congruence and alignment.

Use a range of methods

It is rare for a single teaching method to be universally suitable for all the purposes the teacher has in mind and all the approaches learners may favour. There are very few methods of teaching and, perhaps to a lesser extent, of assessment that are inherently poor. The heart of the matter is selection and appropriate and skilled execution. Much can be done to improve execution – through training, practice, listening to feedback and self-assessment. Selection of methods can also be improved with experience and based on the work of others (see below).

Align choices and focus on the learner (not the teacher)

Unfortunately, and to exaggerate a little, an ineffective approach, at least for complex tasks/materials, has been to transmit some content, think about testing it, set a test, give students a number or grade and consider the task done. An alternative and equally constrained scenario is that of endless student observation of clinical practice with little planned opportunity for hands-on or simulated practice, little conscious structure to help develop reasoning skills, etc. Many readers may recognize the above scenarios as things they experienced during training and may consider that they were no bad thing, enabling them to emerge as successful practitioners. However, other factors have also changed, including an ever more rapid knowledge explosion in the sciences, the increasingly short shelf life of some knowledge, greater requirement for ethical and client-centred practice, and the shortening (at least in medicine) of a lengthy apprentice-style training into a more structured approach.

Suggested approaches for good practice in designing a module or whole curriculum, include:

- Consider the range of knowledge, understanding, skills and attitudes that students need to learn.
- Summarize the most important of these into learning outcomes, which students will be given (at some point), and eventually break them down into objectives for each session.
- Consider the range of teaching and learning methods available and select methods to ensure students will have the opportunity to achieve the outcomes. Rationalize this choice for reasons of efficiency and organization, but retain at least some of the needed features.
- When PBL is the main teaching and learning method, think of teaching and learning methods that will support the PBL, eg, parallel clinical demonstrations that may be needed to fulfil the overall module objectives.
- Consider the learning resources available and align methods of learning and teaching with these.
- 'Design in' giving feedback to students about their progress, and self-assessment. Be aware of the importance to learning of formative assessment.
- Thinking about what the learner needs to achieve and demonstrate, consider how the learning can be assessed (formatively and summatively). Bear in mind that IT may be useful for some methods of assessment, but not a universal panacea.
- Be aware that learning may have valuable consequences that the teacher had not planned for.
- Consider how to offer greater challenge or remediation to those who need it.

Typically, the limiting factors to good practice are resources and timetabling difficulties. Teachers are increasingly exploring how desirable features, from a learning perspective, can be retained under such limiting circumstances. Areas being considered include using IT, peer tutoring, more interactive lectures, etc (see Fry and Marshall, 2001 for more suggestions).

The contrasts between the restricted approach of lectures and MCQs (multiple-choice questions) and good practice suggestions that use a wide range of other approaches, are stark. In the former scenario, assessment is thought of late on in the planning process or is more or less absent, students may be hardly aware of what they are trying to achieve and at best they may think that achievements consist of perfect regurgitation. It is highly unlikely that such a limited approach will assist learners to form desirable attitudes to practice, learn how to communicate with patients, be able to readily use that knowledge when a patient presents with signs and symptoms for diagnosis, be able to process and analyse complex data from a range of sources, cut a cavity, or make a differential diagnosis.

Use evidence, judgement and experience to help make choices

How can a teacher go about selecting compatible teaching methods and forms of assessment? The task is complex, but much help is available. As a starting point, earlier chapters in this book give much good advice. There is also some 'evidence' from robust research about the efficacy of teaching and assessment methods for achieving particular outcomes. However, the use of the research outcomes requires a degree of discrimination – as in education few situations or groups of students are exact replicas of those used in the research. Another source of 'advice' is the experience of self and colleagues about what has worked well in the past. In most instances an element of judgement is involved rather than there being a 'fit all cases' answer.

Learning and teaching using technology

The importance of communications and information technology (C&IT) for the future development of learning and teaching is so great that we revisit it here. Chapter 8 introduced many current developments in the use of C&IT in MDV education and, as identified there, these developments have major implications. In the rush to embrace these new possibilities, the most important issue must be to ensure that the use of C&IT actually improves the student learning experience. The design of courses, their delivery, the range of skills required by learners and by teachers, the composition of teaching teams, quality assurance arrangements, all require a significant shift in our thinking as the full potential of C&IT in education is realized. The challenge is to continue the pedagogical developments that have occurred in higher education and to enhance these with technological developments.

The use of C&IT currently takes many forms in MDV education, ranging from a peripheral to a central component of teaching delivery. As higher education expands it seems inevitable that C&IT will be at the heart of that expansion in the form of online learning. A rapidly growing experience base of online learning and teaching is accumulating, which should inform further developments. The financial resources required to establish and to operate online courses suggest early estimates were optimistic and that this is not a cheap teaching option. Widening the skills base to design and support delivery of courses can take different approaches. The example in Chapter 8 of an online course in teaching and learning in clinical practice, illustrates the composition of a teaching team extending well beyond the 'traditional teacher'. This collaboration does not, however, remove the need for considerable development and training of academic staff. They need support in reconceptualizing how learning takes place and in how to facilitate learning online. Many of us have no personal experience of online learning on which we can draw for our teaching, unlike face-to-face teaching. While many skills used in face-to-face teaching are relevant to online teaching, new ones are required such as the facilitation of asynchronous electronic conference discussions. Institutions pursuing the path of online learning must therefore recognize the need for appropriate staff training.

We believe that the flexibility offered by online learning and teaching is one of the most important features for the expansion of MDV education of all forms – whether for initial training or for continuing professional development. Learners can choose when, where and, sometimes, at what pace they wish to study. For the teacher with a range of other duties, the flexibility of online teaching can seem especially appealing. It is this flexibility that raises the crucial issue of time – time for learning and time for teaching. Students, teachers and managers must recognize the need to allow time for online learning and teaching in the same way that more traditional methods require time. This learning/teaching cannot just be squeezed in around other activities simply because it is flexible, it needs protected time. The classroom helped provide that protection; a current challenge is to devise ways for the virtual classroom to also provide protection for students and teachers alike.

Finally, in exploiting technology, we believe that successful courses must provide for the human element of teaching and learning. New ventures such as the e-University and the NHS university, adopting wholly or partly the use of online learning, can benefit from the substantial experience of the Open University and its attention to the resources to support students learning at a distance, including staff resources. Much of this experience is relevant to online learning. Student motivation is a central aspect of successful learning for which human interaction (whether virtual or real) is required. This, we believe, emphasizes the need for a pedagogic lead for the future successful development of C&IT use in teaching and learning in higher education.

Professional practice

Designing curricula for practice

MDV students have to operate at a great intensity across all the different domains of learning. This may seem daunting but is a feature of students working towards a profession. The GMC, GDC and the RCVS have all emphasized the need for an integrated approach in curriculum design and delivery, bringing together the practice, science and affective elements. Chapter 11 provided an example of the type of change that has been taking place in MDV Schools in recent years – integrating clinical practice into the early stages of the curriculum. Curricula that link different disciplines, that are more learner-centred and that provide the foundation for lifelong learning, are becoming widespread. Problem-based learning lies at the heart of many of these changes. The motivations for such changes are articulated in Chapter 11 and the process of change is well under way. Where then, do the challenges lie for the future?

Chapter 11 identifies three factors for success in starting clinical practice at an early stage of a course:

- the presence of a trusting environment;
- clinical practice based on sound educational theory;
- use of a process of self-reflection and self-assessment.

We consider expanding these factors further. The presence of a trusting environment for students to learn is clearly important if they are to respond to the challenging responsibility placed on them. It is not just the clinical teacher who can create this environment: all stakeholders need to be involved. These include the patients/animal carers, the other staff with whom the student works alongside and, naturally, the students themselves. The clinical teacher has a responsibility to work with these other participants to create the trusting environment. Students need to appreciate and learn the skills for successful interprofessional and patient dialogue and to recognize the changing position of the 'clinical expert' in the provision of MDV care.

Developing skills in self-assessment and reflective practice is central to the aims of preparing students for lifelong learning rather than granting a lifelong licence to practise at the end of a course. Effective self-assessment does not leave all responsibility in the hands of the student; teaching staff need to support the process and provide appropriate feedback. Assessment in general is perhaps one of the areas in which it has proved most challenging to effect change in MDV education. The Quality Assurance Agency identified scope for improvement to various aspects of assessment in its subject overview reports (QAA, 2001), and the GMC explicitly augments its guidance on the matter in its draft recommendations (GMC, 2001). We therefore anticipate further developments in this area, including greater use of self-assessment and peer assessment.

Underlying the success of developing these aspects of clinical teaching is the need to involve all those providing that teaching. Thus, those responsible for teaching the different aspects of clinical practice, science and affective aspects, such as communication skills, need a shared commitment to and understanding of the need for these curricular developments. The importance of team-working skills for students is now well recognized; we should reflect this importance in the way staff work together in providing teaching. Institutional structures and systems do not always facilitate such a shared approach and some rethinking of infrastructure may be necessary and helpful.

Evidence-based practice

More than ever, professionals are under scrutiny and challenge from the public and government. As the new century began, doctors were particularly in the public limelight with widespread media coverage of several high profile cases. Responses include substantial changes to the GMC and its operation. The RCVS notes a growing proportion of graduates involved in claims (RCVS, 2001), while dentists are undergoing similar professional challenge. Partly in response to these changes, the health field has led the way in advocating evidence-based practice. This movement has spawned huge activity in the processing and dissemination of information for practitioners. The Cochrane Collaboration, for example, prepares, maintains and promotes the accessibility of systematic reviews of the effects of healthcare.

Evidence-based practice requires the student to acquire skills in information-seeking and processing, critical appraisal and evaluative judgement. Chapter 8 describes the teaching of information seeking and processing skills integrated into the curriculum rather than as an independent course. Self-help facilities such as the Resource Discovery Network's virtual training suites on accessing bibliographic sources [http://www.vts.rdn.ac.uk/] can support this teaching. Appraisal and evaluation skills can be integrated with the teaching of statistics, for example. A problem-based learning approach can help to foster such skills although it will not automatically generate them; they need explicit attention as much as the subject support does.

It is clear that whatever a student learns as best practice during their course is likely to change over their career. The challenge is to prepare students for using evidence-based practice throughout their professional career and to be prepared to change. Students need guidance, and to develop confidence, in making change to their practice – gauging how much evidence they need, and how to evaluate it. However, this is also true for their teachers. We cannot expect students to acquire these skills if their teachers do not practise them. This implies an openness from teaching staff to the content and the process of their teaching. We consider below some of the challenges ahead:

- In practice, MDV professionals are working with constraints such as financial resources, which lead to ethical and/or political conflicts. For example, evidence directs one to the best drug but this is unaffordable on a widespread basis. Students need to learn how to handle these conflicts in interacting with patients, especially when patients increasingly have access to the same evidence.
- Too great a focus on critical appraisal can lead to overcriticism and rejection of evidence that is perhaps limited but still useful. MDV professionals need to keep a practical perspective but as students they need guidance in making those judgements.
- Debate continues on what constitutes good evidence in terms of matters such as the design of research studies. The position of studies that do not use a randomized controlled trial approach in shaping the evidence base, for example, is hotly disputed (Black, 1996).
- There already exists a vast quantity of information, even in digest form. This demands collaborative work with library and other learning support staff to

guide students and staff to the most useful sources. It also calls for development of infrastructure and preparation of students for instant access to evidence sources that are up-to-date. Facilities that enable a tutor to interact with such sources during a teaching session will be needed.

Ethical practice

One facet of professional behaviour is acting ethically. Since the early 1990s, ethics and law have been accorded gradually more emphasis in the undergraduate curriculum (GMC, 1993 and 2001; GDC, 1997; RCVS, 2001). They are areas of much sensitivity and ambiguity and have regulatory and statutory overtones. Undergraduates, anecdotally, report considerable dissonance between their own values, what they understand to be the values of their profession, what is legal and what they see being practised. Incidents such as the Bristol heart babies case and the Alder Hay organ scandal highlighted the potential need for education for ethical responsibility, and for (self-) monitoring in undergraduate, post-registration and specialist training. Equally important is understanding of the potential ethical implications of differing research designs. In all three professions, ethical and professional behaviour is an aspect of training likely to grow in importance – despite a poor evidence base from which to assume that education can change behaviour and attitudes.

There is increasing interest in the relationship between education and professional values. This is indicated by, for example, increased research on the influence of role models on attitudes. It is also reflected in the use of open discussion groups to ascertain and debate attitudes, of case studies and narratives (eg, see Carson, 2001), and of simulated patients and videoed consultations, to capture and teach about attitude. There has also been interest in how techniques such as moulage (elaborate scenarios to simulate real life) may form and assess behaviour and attitude, or how the collection of opinion on a trainee from members of the team may be used in formal assessment, as long as a large enough sample of views is collected to ensure reliability.

Consideration of ethical practice has also had an impact on professional development outside the education and training arena, eg, in clinical governance, audit and revalidation. The most difficult aspect of this area is that it is no good a student or practitioner knowing what ethical behaviours or legal responsibilities are; what is important is how the registered professional acts in practice.

In the United Kingdom, research is starting to be undertaken on how the training establishment and the early years of clinical contact may influence professional behaviour. The literature of medical education includes a number of recent studies:

- Glasgow Medical School has published on the use of case studies to influence ethical behaviour. They found the skills of the teacher to be crucial (Goldie, Schwartz and Morrison, 2000). They also found vignettes and small groups to be more effective than lecture- and large-group-based teaching for first-year students (Goldie *et al*, 2001). Their work on the teaching and learning of medical ethics in a PBL undergraduate context continues.

- Tulane University Medical School is piloting a programme on Professional Values and Ethics in Medical Education, using a longitudinal approach in which teams of students, residents and faculty form learning teams to address integrity, communication, teamwork, leadership and service. Self- and group reflection is used. Results from the early part of the pilot, using a retreat for first-year medical students to create a learning environment relating to professionalism, indicate some success (Lazarus *et al*, 2000). Evaluation is ongoing.
- The College of Medicine, Texas, has accumulated evidence that moral reasoning skills in medical undergraduates, as measured on a validated, standard instrument can be increased by means of small group case study work, when the period of exposure exceeds 20 hours. Self, Olivarez and Baldwin (1998) conclude that moral reasoning skills are teachable and measurable, but that further work is needed to ascertain generalizability of their findings.
- Educators at Imperial College of Science, Technology and Medicine, London, have collected exercises and documents from a European programme to produce open learning materials for healthcare ethics education. This makes use of experiential learning and uses workbooks for individual or group study. The project aims to develop new models about what should be taught and how (Dickenson and Parker, 1999).

One conclusion that can be drawn from the above is that more undergraduate curriculum time is likely in future to be devoted to ethical practice and that it is likely to be a resource intensive area to teach and monitor. A further implication is the need to continue to train staff in interactive and small group methods of teaching.

Interprofessional practice

All three subjects are becoming more aware of multi- and interprofessional work. As increased emphasis is placed on interprofessionalism (eg, GMC, 2001: 3), education will be important in preparing professionals for changed circumstances of practice, and also be a means by which practice itself will change. Interprofessional refers to members of different professions working together to deliver care and bring about satisfactory outcomes. Examples include, the dental hygienist and dentist; the nurse, surgeon, physiotherapist and occupational therapist; or the vet and veterinary nurse. Purists use interprofessional to refer only to two professions working together, multiprofessional being used for more professions. There are question marks over how far the terms describe teams that work in an integrated manner rather than individuals who liaise about their different spheres of operation.

Interprofessionalism has become increasingly important, as health delivery has blurred some of the roles and distinctions between professionals. It has been suggested that in training, what may be needed is education for working in a team.

Much of this is about communication, flexibility and understanding different roles (Parsell and Bligh, 1999).

There are various ways in which interprofessional education is being addressed. These include having some common or shared teaching, for example, in which trainee members of different professions may be taught together (eg, dental therapist students and dental students), or in which members of different professions learn, in an interactive and supervised environment, how to work with each other to care for patients (Fallsberg and Wijma, 1999; Freeth *et al*, 2000). Many of these activities are fairly early in their development (Horder, 1992) and hard evidence about their efficacy and impact on the quality of patient care is hard to come by. The Medical School of the University of East Anglia is at the forefront of many of these changes.

Changes that merely include joint teaching (eg, sitting in lectures) may do little to change attitudes. Parsell and Bligh (1999) found overcoming structural and organizational difficulties hard, but less difficult than changing attitudes. Issues under considerable scrutiny concern the timing (eg, early in the curriculum before professional socialization, or later so as to create less confusion about role) of such intervention and the teaching and learning methods to be used. Another aspect is the need for staff development for those who will teach or supervise interprofessional education. It can be expected that the early years of the 21st century will see the collection of considerably more information about the efficacy of different approaches to interprofessional education, as well as an increased emphasis from regulatory bodies.

Lifelong learning

A seamless education?

Education and training for the three professions in the mid- to late-twentieth century tended to reinforce boundaries between under- and postgraduate training. The norm was for little continuity, with little thought given to the transition from student to fully fledged professional. That position is changing. The exact registration regulations for each profession vary, but the taking of a more 'holistic' view of training and professional registration and practice is common. In medicine, the expression a 'sixth year' is increasingly used, as deanery and university work in greater cooperation. In dentistry, the postgraduation and registration year is increasingly being monitored so that the legal position of being able to undertake independent practice still obtains, but the reality is of some continuing supervision, education and training. Veterinary medicine looks set to adopt a similar position (RCVS, 2001). In the last year of undergraduate education there is increasing emphasis on practice, with many newer curricula featuring shadowing of PRHOs (pre-registration house officers), or equivalent, integrated dental practice for final year students and so on.

These features have implications for teaching and curriculum organization. They reinforce the message that curricula should do more than focus on content. They place emphasis on teaching and supervision by and from practising professionals and imply graduates with considerable practical competence (especially in dental and veterinary medicine). These features should reduce barriers between training establishments and the deliverers of healthcare. A further change has been a more structured approach to consideration of the knowledge and skills that need to be acquired post-registration.

The burdens for the professions, and hence for teachers, are matched only by the complexity of the task. Those teaching undergraduates in the three professions need training in basic teaching methods, but also in assessment, and in how to design curricula that take account of the contemporary practice of medicine, dentistry and veterinary science. Effective organization and management of the resulting complex curricula and post-registration arrangements are key; and often neglected. In terms of this volume, the portions of the assessment chapter on standard setting, feedback and clinical and personal skills, and the chapters on supporting students and learning in the clinical environment will be particularly useful.

Progress files

A progress file is a mix of a record of achievement and a workbook for reflecting on learning and career development. The term 'progress file' originated with the *Dearing Report* into higher education (Dearing, 1997) and was elaborated by the Quality Assurance Agency (QAA, 2000). Each higher education institution has been counselled to develop its own model of a progress file; they may be more or less sensitive to their use in the medical, dental and veterinary professions.

Progress files represent a considerable opportunity for the three subject areas, individually or jointly, to draw together a number of distinctive features of their education. These include logbooks, reflections on practice such as journals and diaries, self-assessment, and official records about the options and grades obtained during a university qualification. Many of these devices have been referred to earlier in this book, but the progress file offers an opportunity for their integration, for use across a team, and for thinking about using these tools on a lifelong basis to enhance career planning, updating, continuous professional development and recertification (see for example Fry *et al*, 2002).

The medical first degree at Manchester has developed a progress file to promote reflection on learning, particularly in relation to special study modules, others focus on clinical practice, some are paper-based and some delivered mainly through an electronic medium. It is vital that MDV education considers how progress files can be integrated into other arrangements and used to achieve ends central to professional practice and lifelong learning.

Continuing professional development (CPD) and recertification

This chapter and earlier ones have referred to the need for MDV professionals to be prepared for lifelong learning – for updating their knowledge and skills, for changing their practice on the basis of new evidence. Equally important is acquiring and retaining the skills and attitudes needed for lifelong learning – the package of approaches often called 'learning to learn'. A more seamless pathway through undergraduate and postgraduate study, the shift to student-centred learning, the introduction of self-assessment and support for reflective practice, and the introduction of progress files are some of the opportunities for this preparation.

MDV professionals will increasingly require opportunities for further development and for diverse ways of obtaining these opportunities, many of which will require input from academics and leading practitioners. One challenge for CPD is how to move on from it being little more than a box-ticking exercise. How can we best motivate professionals for further learning and provide opportunities that are congruent with busy professional lives?

Busy professionals cannot absent themselves for study on the same basis as full-time undergraduates. Many professional societies and colleges now accredit activities such as discussion meetings and workshops as well as more formal courses. The keeping of portfolios and the videoing of practice are also coming to the fore. Other activities such as study trips to centres (or persons) of excellence will also need to be accredited and encouraged. As discussed earlier in this chapter, technology can help to provide study flexibility, although this requires new skills and approaches and supporting resources. Assessment, appraisal and monitoring will come to the fore, and events will go full circle with the need, already recognized by the GMC and alluded to earlier in this chapter, for undergraduates to become accustomed to this climate of appraisal, professional updating and responsibility.

Those faced with today's undergraduates also need to support yesterday's graduates in updating their learning. Separation of new and 'returning learners' may not always be the best way forward and we should look at ways to maximize the benefits and limit the difficulties of mixing the two groups. The returning learners clearly have a lot to offer the undergraduate from their actual experience, which may be more current than that of the teacher. Undergraduates can bring fresh insights to old problems and often possess better skills in areas such as IT, which they can share with the experienced professional. Both parties, and any tutors involved, are likely to need introduction to working successfully in this way.

Conclusion

In the preceding sections we have attempted to identify some of the future pathways and challenges facing MDV education. We conclude with some closing remarks on their implications for staff and institutions. An obvious implication is the need for educational development and training of staff to support them in making the types of change indicated above. If institutions and employers are to deliver on the demands of the public, the Royal Colleges and the statutory bodies, then they will have to be prepared to support their staff and provide facilities for study and development opportunities and make provision for the costs entailed.

Supporting these needs is at the heart of recent initiatives such as the Institute for Learning and Teaching and the establishment of the Learning and Teaching Support Network of Subject Centres. Such bodies aim to assist in improved dissemination of good practice in teaching and in promoting the need for greater priority to be attached to training and teaching in higher education. Their success or otherwise depends, however, on participation from across the sector, helping to set the agenda and identify support needs.

Institutions face growing pressure on their resources as they attempt to meet the increasingly complex demands on their education and training provision. In addition to the support and development of staff, review of structural and organizational aspects need attention to tackle more effectively issues such as integrated curricula and interprofessional teaching. It is fashionable, and many would say trite, to say that institutions must be aware of the global platform on which they increasingly operate. Nevertheless, failure to be aware of and to prepare for the changing nature of higher education in the United Kingdom and elsewhere could cost institutions dearly. How far, for example, will developments such as the e-university and the NHS university complement or detract from existing provision in the MDV field?

Current developments in MDV education have been informed by research, although it is arguable to what extent. As the pressure to meet the challenging agendas increases, more research is needed to establish a better evidence base for further developments. In a subject field where evidence-based practice is already prevalent, we believe staff will respond more readily to make changes in teaching and learning where there is clear evidence to support the changes. A positive step would be to attach greater recognition to the value of such research in order to encourage participation from those involved in the practice. This recognition needs to occur at institutional level and at national level. For example, debates on how the Research Assessment Exercise recognizes such research require continuing development.

Finally, this book comprises contributions and examples from across the three areas of MDV education. Unsurprisingly, there are many similarities in the issues that each area is facing and the developments that are occurring. We hope, however, that the reader from one of these areas will have found food for thought in the experiences of another and be encouraged to seek greater sharing of practice as further developments occur.

References

Black, N (1996) Why we need observational studies to evaluate the effectiveness of health care, *British Medical Journal*, **312** (7040), pp 1215–18

Carson, A M (2001) That's another story: narrative methods and ethical practice, *Journal of Medical Ethics*, **27** (3), pp 198–202

Dearing, R (1997) *Report of the National Committee of Inquiry into Higher Education*, Chapter 9: 20 [Online] http://www.leeds.ac.uk/educol/ncihe/

Dickenson, D and Parker, M (1999) The European Biomedical Ethics Practitioner Education Project: an experiential approach to philosophy and ethics in health care education, *Medicine, Health Care and Philosophy*, **2** (3), pp 231–37

Fallsberg, M and Wijma, K (1999) Student Attitudes towards the goals of an Interprofessional Training Ward, *Medical Teacher*, **21**, pp 576–81

Freeth, M *et al* (2000) Education for clinical governance: an interprofessional approach, *Journal of Interprofessional Care*, **14**, pp 292–93

Fry, H *et al* (2002) Developing Progress Files: a case study, *Teaching in Higher Education*, **7** (1), pp 99–113

Fry, H and Marshall, S (2001) Revitalizing and Renewing the Curriculum, in *The Effective Academic*, eds S Ketteridge, S Marshall and H Fry, Kogan Page, London

GDC (General Dental Council) (1997) *The First Five Years*, GDC, London

GDC (2002) *Lifelong Learning* [Online] http://www.gdcuk.org/lifelong/LifeLongLearning.htm

GMC (1993) *Tomorrow's Doctors*, GMC, London

GMC (1995) *Duties of a Doctor*, GMC, London

GMC (2001) *Draft Recommendations on Undergraduate Medical Education*, GMC, London

GMC (2002) *Web reference pages for recertification* [Online] http://www.gmcuk.org/revalidation/html

Goldie, J G S, Schwartz, L, Morrison, J M (2000) A process evaluation of medical ethics education in the first year of a new medical curriculum, *Medical Education*, **34**, pp 468–73

Goldie J, Schwartz, L, McConnachie, A, Morrison, J (2001) Impact of a new course on students' potential behaviour on encountering ethical dilemmas, *Medical Education*, **35**, pp 295–302

Horder, J (1992) A national survey that needs to be repeated, *Journal of Interprofessional Care*, **6**, pp 65–71

Lazarus, C *et al* (2000) The program for professional values and ethics in medical education, *Teaching and Learning in Medicine*, **12** (4), pp 208–11

Parsell, G and Bligh, J (1999) The development of a questionnaire to assess the readiness of health care students for interprofessional learning (RIPLS), *Medical Education*, **33** (2), pp 95–100

Quality Assurance Agency (QAA) (2000) *Developing a Progress File for Higher Education*, QAA, London

QAA (2001) *Subject review overview reports for Medicine, Dentistry and Veterinary Medicine* [Online] http://www.qaa.ac.uk/revreps/subjrev/intro.htm

Ramsden, P (1992) *Learning to Teach in Higher Education*, Routledge, London

RCVS (Royal College of Veterinary Surgeons) (2001) *Veterinary Education and Training. A Framework for 2010 and Beyond*, RCVS, London

Self, D, Olivarez, M and Baldwin, D J (1998) The amount of small-group case-study discussion needed to improve moral reasoning skills of medical students, *Academic Medicine*, **73** (5), pp 521–23

Index